Traditional Chinese Medicine

Traditional Chinese Medicine

Oliver Frakes

SYRAWOOD
PUBLISHING HOUSE

New York

Published by Syrawood Publishing House,
750 Third Avenue, 9th Floor,
New York, NY 10017, USA
www.syrawoodpublishinghouse.com

Traditional Chinese Medicine
Oliver Frakes

International Standard Book Number: 978-1-64740-016-3 (Hardback)

Cataloging-in-Publication Data

Traditional chinese medicine / Oliver Frakes.
    p. cm.
Includes bibliographical references and index.
ISBN 978-1-64740-016-3
1. Medicine, Chinese. 2. Alternative medicine. 3. Medicine. I. Frakes, Oliver.
R601 .T73 2020
610.951--dc23

TABLE OF CONTENTS

PREFACE

The branch of traditional medicine which is based on ancient Chinese medical practices is known as Traditional Chinese Medicine or TCM. There are various forms of medicine which are considered to be a part of TCM such as cupping therapy, bonesetter, gua sha, acupuncture and herbal medicine. The primary belief of TCM is that the body's vital energy, which is also called chi, circulates through channels, which are called meridians. The functions of the body such as breathing and digestion are the primary focus of this branch of medicine, instead of the anatomical structures. This book provides significant information of this discipline to help develop a good understanding of Traditional Chinese medicine and related fields. Some of the diverse topics covered in it address the varied branches that fall under this category. This book is appropriate for students seeking detailed information in this area as well as for experts.

A short introduction to every chapter is written below to provide an overview of the content of the book:

Chapter 1 - The branch of traditional medicine which was conceived in China is termed as traditional Chinese medicine. Some of the major theories within it are yinyang theory and five phase theory. This is an introductory chapter which will introduce briefly all the diverse aspects of traditional Chinese medicine such as its healing modalities and therapeutic principles; **Chapter 2 -** The model of the body according to traditional Chinese medicine consists of numerous components such as qi, xue, jinye, zang fu and jing luo. The topics elaborated in this chapter will help in gaining a better perspective about these components as well as the relationships between essence, qi, blood and body fluids; **Chapter 3 -** The branch of traditional Chinese medicine which makes use of plant elements as well as animal, human and mineral products for the treatment of ailments is termed as Chinese herbology. The diverse applications of Chinese herbology for the purpose of qi-regulation, heat clearing and phlegm resolution have been thoroughly discussed in this chapter; **Chapter 4 -** The branch of traditional Chinese medicine which involves the insertion of needles into the body is termed as acupuncture. Moxibustion refers to a form of therapy within Chinese traditional medicine where dried mugwort is burned on specific point of the body. The topics elaborated in this chapter will help in gaining a better perspective about moxibustion as well as the different practices within acupuncture such as auricular acupuncture and electroacupuncture; **Chapter 5 -** The diagnosis in traditional Chinese medicine makes use of numerous diagnostic methods, such as the examination of the tongue and the pulse. This chapter closely examines the key concepts related to these diagnostic methods in traditional Chinese medicine as well as the eight principles of diagnosis to provide an extensive understanding of the subject; **Chapter 6 -** There are various therapies which are used within traditional Chinese medicine. A few of them are Chinese cupping, Chinese tuina massage, gua sha, acupressure, qi gong, tai chi and Chinese dietary therapy. This chapter has been carefully written to provide an easy understanding of the varied facets of these therapies in traditional Chinese medicine.

I extend my sincere thanks to the publisher for considering me worthy of this task. Finally, I thank my family for being a source of support and help.

Oliver Frakes

Chapter 1

Traditional Chinese Medicine: An Introduction

The branch of traditional medicine which was conceived in China is termed as traditional Chinese medicine. Some of the major theories within it are Yinyang theory and five phase theory. This is an introductory chapter which will introduce briefly all the diverse aspects of traditional Chinese medicine such as its healing modalities and therapeutic principles.

Traditional Chinese medicine (TCM) is one of the most established systems of medicine in the world. The therapeutic formulae used in TCM are frequently derived from aqueous decoctions of single plants or complex multicomponent formulae. There are aspects of plant cultivation and preparation of decoction pieces that are unique to TCM. These include Daodi cultivation, which is associated with high quality medicinal plant material that is grown in a defined geographical area, and Paozhi processing where the decoction pieces can be treated with excipients and are processed, which may fundamentally change the nature of the chemical metabolites. Therefore, a single plant part, processed in a variety of different ways, can each create a unique medicine. The quality of TCM materials, their safety and therapeutic efficacy are of critical importance. The application of metabolomic and chemometric techniques to these complex and multicomponent medicines is of interest to understand the interrelationships between composition, synergy and therapeutic activity.

Traditional Chinese medicine (TCM) has been used extensively for thousands of years and is the initial medical treatment that the ancient Chinese used to treat wounds and diseases. With the passage of time, Chinese people began to investigate and record the pharmacological activities of the herbs they were using, based on experience. They classified medicinal herbs into five flavours which are pungent, sweet, sour, bitter and salty, forming the earliest system in TCM. As Confucianism and Taoism developed, yin and yang, the five elements (metal, wood, water, fire and earth) and the seven-relation compatibility were introduced and incorporated into TCM. These concepts influenced the development of TCM treatments and therapeutic formulae called Fangji. Fangji are composed of multiple herbs with integrated medical effects and are guided by the concepts underpinning TCM.

Herbal materials used in TCM are often extracted with water to make an aqueous extract or decoction. Single herbs, or multiple herbs combined in one formula, can be used to make multicomponent TCMs. Multicomponent therapeutic formulae are the most important and are most commonly used in TCM for clinical applications. The extraction methods employed to produce aqueous decoctions can vary, depending on the different compositions of the formulae. The details of the extraction methods are important as the methodology can impact the chemicals extracted, and hence, the therapeutic effect of the decoction.

As for all herbal medicinal products (HMPs), the therapeutic effects of TCM are influenced by many factors which affect the quality of the starting materials, for example, quality and age of seed stock, climate, soil, humidity, temperature and sunlight. Factors such as storage, contamination and pollutants can also affect the quality of materials. For TCM, there are some unique traditional practices that can determine the therapeutic activity of the materia medica. These notably include specific cultivation, harvesting, fumigation and processing methods of fresh herbal material, which are keys to the quality, efficacy and safety of TCM.

'Materia medica' for TCM decoctions is described as Daodi when cultivated under particular conditions in specific geographic regions and processed with specific methods. In TCM, Daodi medicine is recognised as meeting the highest quality standards and denotes superior clinical properties. Modern scientific research supports the fact that Daodi medicinal herbs are more potent than non-Daodi grown samples of the same herb. The second key term in the production of TCM is Paozhi, which is defined as a group of methods for preparing TCM to generate material with different clinical or therapeutic purposes. Paozhi methods are guided by TCM theory, and their use differentiates TCM from western herbal medicine. For example, the same herb can be processed in different ways, and Shan zha (*Crataegi fructus*), a fruit, is usually fried. This process results in fruit with the generic term 'Chao'. Different approaches to process the fruit yield different Chao, including Yellow Chao, Charred Chao and Carbonised Chao. The decoctions that result from the different forms of Chao are different in terms of chemical composition, and the resulting decoctions are used to treat different degrees of intestinal disease. Furthermore, processing methods are also very important for the safety and storage of TCM and have a direct impact on the consistency and quality of the Chinese herbal medicine. In general, the variations in quality, safety and efficacy in TCM are the most significant barriers faced by China in gaining access for TCM into European and North-American markets.

Currently, sustainability of ecological resources is attracting global attention, especially for medicinal herbal plants. Since they are in large demand in Asian countries and natural products are gaining in popularity in the European and American markets, there is a major challenge relating to sustainable supply of herbal materials. Thus, cultivation is being adopted to solve the problems caused by wild harvesting.

Nowadays, as modern analytical techniques become more sensitive and metabolomic methodologies become more refined, chemometric analysis of TCM is used to investigate the relationship between chemical profiles, candidate components and bioactivities. Multiple methods, such as hyphenated chromatographic and spectroscopic techniques (e.g., liquid chromatography-mass spectrometry (LC-MS), gas chromatography-mass spectrometry (GC-MS) and liquid chromatography-nuclear magnetic resonance (LC-NMR)) are applied to determine the chemical fingerprints and to correlate these with bioactivities of TCM. Chemometric techniques advance our understanding of composition and bioactivity of extracts and include, among others, principal component analysis (PCA), linear discriminate analysis (LDA), spectral correlative chromatography (SCC) and information theory (IT).

The guidance of TCM theory for the generation of Paozhi and therapeutic formulae impacts the chemical composition and final therapeutic effects of medicinal herbs. In contrast, phytomedicine focuses on identification and isolation of individual chemical components, lacking the characteristics of Fangji in traditional Chinese medicine theory, where herbal formulae are organised using the Jun-Chen-Zuo-Shi system. Combining the pharmacological analysis of multiple biomarkers with chemical fingerprint analysis can help to provide an understanding of how the therapeutic effect of herbal formulae is produced.

More recently, modern formulations of traditional TCM decoctions have come on the market. These involve the formation of granulated material, by combining decoctions with excipients and subjecting them to spray drying and granulation to create stable products. Such dried decoction material can also be incorporated into capsules. Modernised TCM formulations are more easily transported and stored and can have a long shelf life than the original herbal material. Some commonly-used TCMs have been formulated in such a way. However, the efficacy of these emerging, modernised TCM formulations has not been fully evaluated by international researchers. In addition, solving the efficacy equivalence between decoction pieces and new formulations is an important problem for the modernisation of TCM.

Therefore, TCM is the final product of several complex factors, that is, TCM theory, medicinal herbs, modern formulations and modern research as detailed in figure.

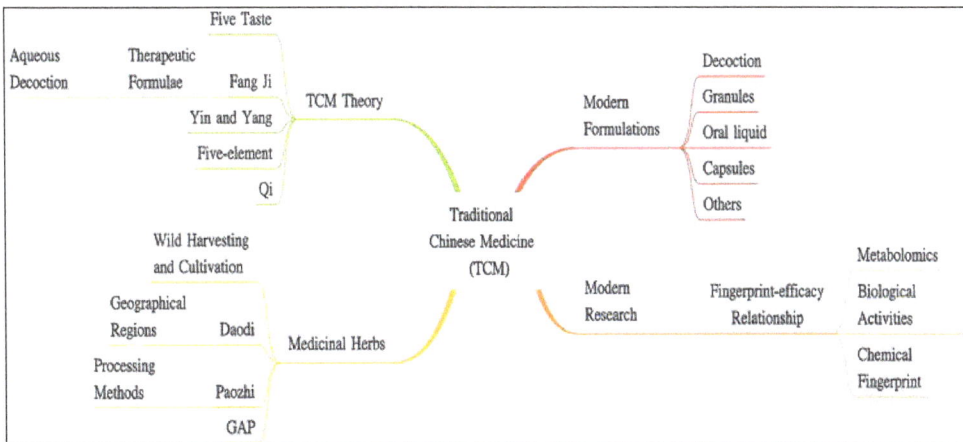

Main factors that contribute to modern TCM.

From Aqueous Extracts to Therapeutic Formulae

Decoction of herbs, the most important preparation method of Chinese medicine, was first invented and further developed between 2000 and 474 BC. The medical ingredients were extracted by boiling in water or alcohol, with special preparation times that depend on the properties of the ingredients. Following this, the decoction was filtered, and the resulting liquid was taken by patients. In modern China, the method of decoction is still the most commonly used process in TCM.

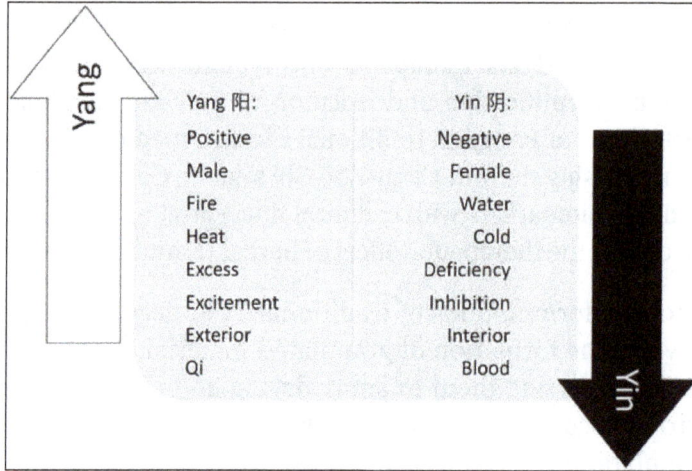

Yin and Yang theory.

In TCM, most of the disease diagnosis and principles of medical application are based on a particular Chinese philosophy that is aligned with Confucianism and Taoism. The theory of TCM refers to Yin and Yang, the five elements, zangfu, channels-collaterals, qi, blood, body fluids, methods of diagnosis, differentiation of symptom-complexes, etc. Yin and Yang are opposite and complementary sides of the nature in the universe, and, according to Chinese philosophy, everything could be described by Yin and Yang. In TCM, Yin refers to the material aspects of the organism, and Yang refers to functions. It is the interpretation that the disease is caused by the imbalance of Yin and Yang in the human body. The rationale of Chinese medicine is to bring Yin and Yang back into balance, which results in overall health and cure versus the disease.

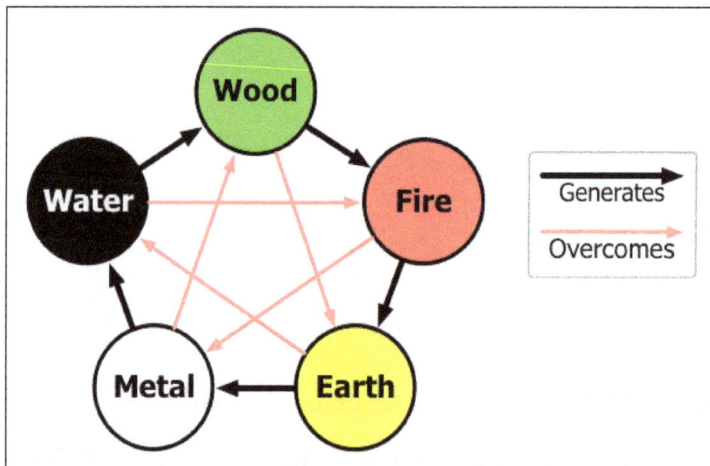

The principle of the five elements system.

In addition, in ancient Chinese theory, everything in the universe consists of five elements (metal, wood, water, fire and earth). All organs and tissues were assigned to different elements, which are differentiated by their properties. This is the special Chinese system theory that forms a basis for TCM. Chinese medicine is very different from Western medicine, and the methodology of disease treatment cannot be explained in the same way as in modern medicine, as it is a type of treatment that is based on experience and a special philosophy.

After the 1950s, advanced research into TCM began, which was aimed at meeting the needs of the growing Chinese population and also at reaching the standards of safety, efficacy and quality of Western medicine. In the 1970s, Youyou Tu was inspired by a book about TCM, the 'Zhou-Hou-Bei-Ji-Fang' (317–420 AD), in which *Artemisia carvifolia* (Qing hao) was described as being extracted with water to produce a decoction, and this was used to treat malaria symptoms. This led her to isolate artemisinin from the Qing hao plant. Artemisinin was successfully tested for the treatment of epidemic diseases including malaria in China, which ultimately led to Youyou Tu to being awarded the Nobel Prize in 2015.

With the passage of time, TCM was also delivered in increasingly diverse formulations, other than decoctions, such as wines, pills and plasters. Currently, modernised formulae such as granules, oral liquids, capsules, dissolved medicines and ointments are coming onto the market. These modern formulations are produced by a small number, currently six, of State approved pharmaceutical industries. China introduced the concept of 'internationalization of TCM' in 1996, to address sustainable production and to promote export and international trading, and as a result, the quality, safety and regulatory requirements for TCM have gained increasing international attention and have promoted the formation of international consortia working to this end.

Daodi Herbal Medicine

Daodi is a term unique to TCM and is reserved for medicinal plants cultivated in a specific geographical area with specified natural conditions and being harvested and processed following standards. 'Dao' refers to the measurement unit of districts in ancient China, and 'di' refers to earth, land or soil. It is stated in an ancient materia medica 'Xin-Xiu-Ben-Cao' that the medical efficacy will be different if the medicinal material is not grown in its native environment. Daodi medical material has been regarded as superior medicine for centuries and is recognised as such by today's TCM pharmaceutical industry. The Daodi material is more vibrant and less dense. In the Chinese Pharmacopoeia, 284 different kinds of TCM plant materials are recognised to have Daodi specifications from a total of 584 commonly used medicinal plants.

TCM knowledge and expertise have grown over millennia of clinical experience, resulting in the discovery and understanding of the differing properties of herbal material, which depend on their quality, and often are impacted by the source.

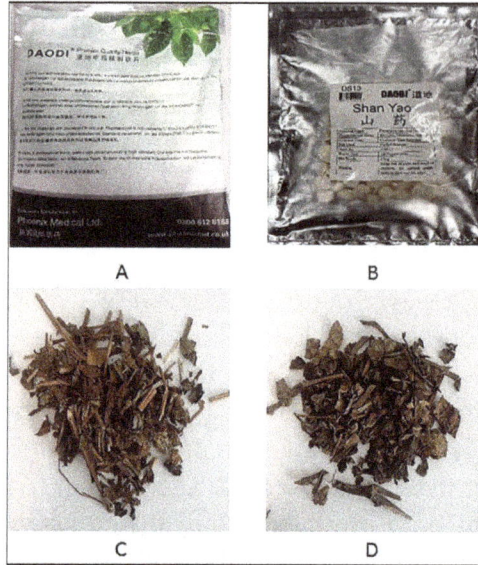

Commercial TCM products: (A) Houttuynia cordata (Yu xing cao). (B) Radix Dioscoreae oppositae (Shan yao). (C) Daodi Houttuynia cordata decoction pieces. (D) Non-Daodi Houttuynia cordata decoction pieces.

The characteristics of plants are determined by genetics; however, the diverse landforms and weather in China resulted in different ecosystems, which contributed to a variety of botanical germ plasm origins. Additionally, specific ecological conditions such as topography, soil, climate, humidity and light also influenced the number of secondary metabolites of plants, which resulted in different bioactivities of a particular herbal material. Therefore, the combination of the geographical location and the specific germ plasm resulted in the superior quality of the Daodi medical material.

In the first modern monograph of Daodi medicinal material in the Chinese Pharmacopoeia, 159 different medicinal materials are classified into 8 categories according to the various production regions in China: Chuan (Sichuan), Guang (Guang dong/Guang xi), Yun (Yun nan), Gui (Gui zhou), Nan (Southern China), Bei (Northern China), Zhe (Zhe jiang) and Huai (He nan). Interesting examples include *Liguisticum chuanxiong* Hort. (Chuan xiong), which belongs to Chuan Daodi medica material, because the Sichuan province is the native region for cultivation and is known to have the largest output and longest history of medical application of Chuan xiong. *Liguisticum chuanxiong* Hort. cv. *Fuxiong* (Fu xiong) is produced in the Jiangxi province and has large and fleshy rhizomes similar to Daodi Chuan Xiong; however, it has been shown that it contained less essential oil by chemical analysis, which resulted in different bioactivities. Ginseng is one of the most famous and expensive TCM plant materials, and the Daodi production region of ginseng is in North-Eastern China. In 1958, ginseng was cultivated on the Hailan island in Southern China, which resulted in large roots which were lacking bioactive constituents. In the past 10 years, chemical constituents of volatile oil in the rhizomes and radices of *Notopterygium incisum* Ting (Qiang huo) from different regions were investigated by GC. In the Sichuan Daodi sample, 769 compounds were identified and quantified and showed significant differences in the chemical composition of samples that were produced in other non-Daodi geographical regions.

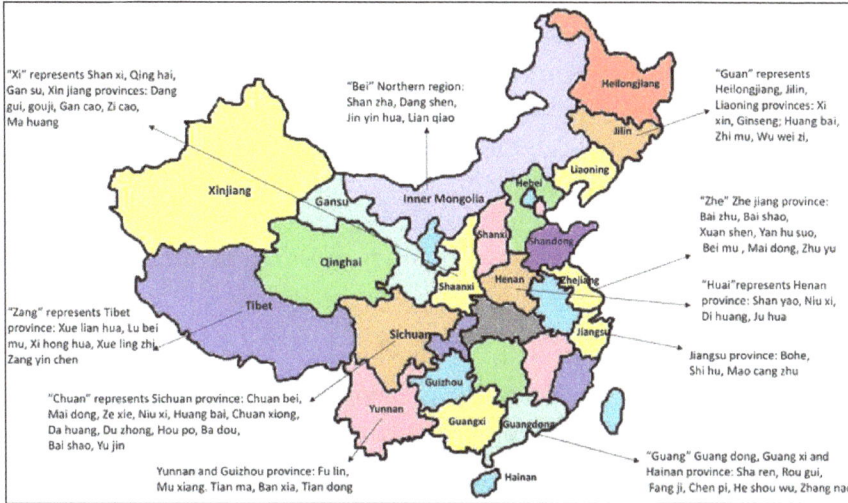

"Xi" represents Shan xi, Qing hai, Gan su, Xin jiang provinces: Dang gui, gouji, Gan cao, Zi cao, Ma huang

"Bei" Northern region: Shan zha, Dang shen, Jin yin hua, Lian qiao

"Guan" represents Heilongjiang, Jilin, Liaoning provinces: Xi xin, Ginseng; Huang bai, Zhi mu, Wu wei zi,

"Zhe" Zhe jiang province: Bai zhu, Bai shao, Xuan shen, Yan hu suo, Bei mu , Mai dong, Zhu yu

"Huai"represents Henan province: Shan yao, Niu xi, Di huang, Ju hua

"Zang" represents Tibet province: Xue lian hua, Lu bei mu, Xi hong hua, Xue ling zhi, Zang yin chen

Jiangsu province: Bohe, Shi hu, Mao cang zhu

"Chuan" represents Sichuan province: Chuan bei, Mai dong, Ze xie, Niu xi, Huang bai, Chuan xiong, Da huang, Du zhong, Hou po, Ba dou, Bai shao, Yu jin

Yunnan and Guizhou province: Fu lin, Mu xiang. Tian ma, Ban xia, Tian dong

"Guang" Guang dong, Guang xi and Hainan province: Sha ren, Rou gui, Fang ji, Chen pi, He shou wu, Zhang nao

Map of Daodi medicines produced in 10 regions in China.

Nowadays, with the increased need for herbal medicines for health purposes, including food supplements, nutraceuticals and skincare products, it is recognised that the Daodi region cannot produce sufficient plant materials to meet the market demand. Since 2002, the Chinese government is emphasising Good Agricultural Practice (GAP) for the cultivation of medicinal materials, which is aimed at expanding the production regions. According to the Good practice of TCM report of the European commission in 2012, Daodi medicinal herbs and also new Daodi medicines will be allowed to emerge. For instance, Daodi *Radix Salviae miltiorrhizae* (Dan shen) that was cultivated exclusively in Sichuan, is now produced on large-scale standardised plantations in the non-Daodi region Shanxi province by modern TCM pharmaceutical companies. The Tasly pharmaceutical company was the first, approved by GAP, in China for the large-scale standardised plantation. Goji (fruits of *Lycium barbarum* L. and *Lycium chinense* Mill), which has been applied in TCM treatment for millennia to treat imbalance of yin, is now experiencing an increased demand as it is also seen as 'super food' and recommended as potent antioxidant in the Western world. The Ningxia province is recognised as the Daodi region for Goji, but the increasing market led to new cultivations in other regions such as in the Hubei, Qinghai and Xinjiang province, where the geographical and climatic conditions are different to the Daodi region. Goji produced from those regions also has very high quality, but is different in the number of metabolites, such as polysaccharides, flavonoids, betaine and carotenoids. Therefore, it is still challenging to achieve the aim of GAP. In Yao's group, the antioxidant activities of Daodi Goji and non-Daodi Goji were studied, and the IC50 values of the radical-scavenging effect for both Goji treatment groups were determined to be even higher than the positive control group which was treated by Quercetin.

Daodi medicinal material plays an essential role in TCM treatment, but its superior quality has not yet been adequately explained by modern science. Comparisons between Daodi and non-Daodi materials have been studied mainly in terms of bioactive ingredients or composition, soil properties, the geological background system (GBS) and some identification methodologies to assess Daodi attributes, which might be closely related to bioactive ingredient production. However, the superior quality, safety and efficacy of Daodi products still remain to be investigated. Current research of Daodi products focuses on the identification and authentication of species in the Daodi region, establishment and implementation of the commercial specification criteria and standardisation of plantation and processing. Therefore, there is a need for further research in TCM to establish many factors that influence the potency of Daodi medical material.

Cultivation versus Wild Harvesting

China is reported to have the largest number of medicinal herbs, with approximately 11,146 being used in 2016. TCM is based on wild medicinal herbs resources, and it was stated in 2015 that they account for approximately 80% of the total Chinese herbs resources. To meet the increasingly higher demands from the domestic and global market and also to achieve the sustainable utilisation of medicinal herbs, some scale-up cultivation projects for TCM herbs have been established. Moreover, natural foresting, which is closer to wild harvesting but different to conservative artificial cultivation, is recommended to be applied for production of some medicinal herbs, such as *Fritillaria cirrhosa* (Chuan bei mu), *Radix Ginseng* (Ren shen) and Huang lian, *but* the cost is much higher than that of cultivation. It is anticipated that cultivation of medicinal herbs will satisfy the market demand and reduce the ecological pressure caused by wild harvesting. Outcomes for cultivation show that it is an approach suited to some herbal material, and the appearance and efficacy are very close to herbs harvested wildly. However, high upfront costs can be associated with the construction of the special environment needed for mass cultivation, but the economic and ecological benefits of cultivation versus wild harvesting are recognised.

However, the consistent quality of herbs from artificial cultivation and wild harvesting is still a challenge for most TCM herbs, because quality, safety and efficacy of medicinal herbs can be impacted by variations in cultivation. For example, the active components of *Ranunculus ternatus* are polysaccharides, and the concentration of which varies significantly between samples collected by natural fostering and wild collection, 10 and 14%, respectively. To solve the problems of artificial cultivation, standard operating procedures, which include germ plasm selection, breeding, fertilisation, irrigation, pest control and limitation of toxic substances, are required to improve the quality of TCM close to that of the wild harvested herbs.

Cultivation and wild harvesting have advantages and disadvantages. For cultivation, soil fertility has a significant impact on the yield of the major chemical components in herbal materials, and the lack of standards for soil fertility will result in unsure biomass and quality of medicinal herb production. The standards for soil fertility should include soil texture, density, moisture content, soil acidity, nitrogen and phosphorus content and microorganisms. For wild harvesting, the quality of medicinal herbs is determined by factors such as identification, time of harvesting, harvesting methods and transportation. Harvesting methods should avoid damage to harvested material and to surrounding herbs. The ideal quantity of harvested herbal material should be scientifically considered and balanced, to allow for sustainability. The period of harvesting is important as the effective chemical contents of herbs vary seasonally and climatically, which will impact on biological activity of the decoctions derived from the herbal material.

Wild harvesting can be considered 'treasure from the nature', as the material comes from the natural resource without the addition of pesticides. Furthermore, for most of medicinal herbs, wild harvested material is superior, with resultant decoctions being more potent. However, overloaded harvesting causes an imbalance in the ecological environment and threatens the quantities of wild resource of especially rare or endangered species. Codonopsis pilosula (Dang shen), Dan shen, Radix isatidis seu Baphcacanthi (Ban lan gen), ginseng and Coptis chinensis (Huang lian) are some of the key TCM herbs cultivated in different regions in China. Without doubt, the management policy and practice of wild harvesting of natural resources require further development, if goals of sustainable supply of this resource are to be achieved.

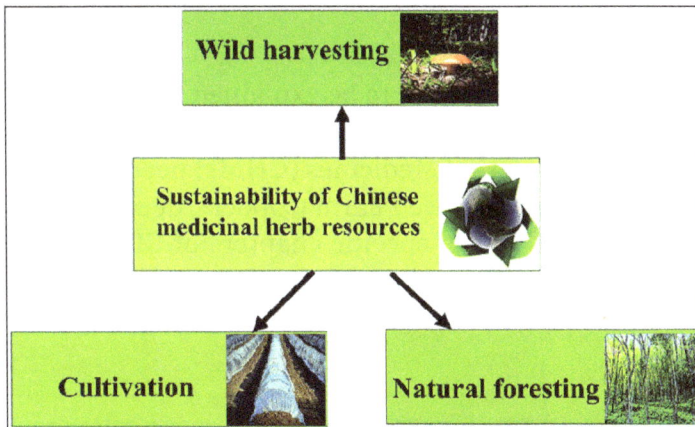

Wild harvesting, natural foresting and cultivation contribute
to the sustainability of Chinese medicinal herb resources.

The cultivation of medicinal plant material reduces the ecological impact caused by extensive wild-harvesting and can also protect the standardised genotypes of species, contributing to the sustainable production and utilisation of Chinese medicinal herbs. Cultivation also has an economic benefit, with new industries and employment models emerging, and guaranteeing the supply for the expanding and substantial Chinese and global markets. However, one negative impact is that the natural diversity of the gene pool for wild resources is reducing due to the standardisation of mass cultivation practices. A reasonable balance of cultivation, wild harvesting and natural foresting will ultimately be the best model and will contribute to the sustainability of TCM herb resources.

Paozhi

Paozhi is a unique traditional processing technique, which differentiates TCM from Western herbal medicine. The processed products following Paozhi are known as decoction pieces. With the guidance of TCM theory and according to the properties of medicinal plants, the raw herbal medicine is processed to suit the TCM therapeutic purpose. In TCM theory, it is the belief that disease is caused by the imbalance of Yin and Yang, and ancient Chinese people believe that the processing procedure could adjust the 'Qi' (heat, warm, cold and cool qualities) of raw herbal medicines, to equilibrate the balance of Yin and Yang in the human body.

Processing methods are usually different for different medicinal plants, and this is due to the nature of the material, for example, radix (root), rhizoma (rhizome or lateral root), herba (herb, whole plant) and flos (flower) and the purpose for their clinical application. The main aim of Paozhi is to enhance the efficacy and reduce toxicity. For instance, Radix Aconiti kusnezofii (Cao Wu tou) is processed to reduce toxicity for safe use by steaming or boiling with Radix glycyrrhizae (Gan cao) and Semen Sojae hispidae (Hei dou). Paozhi is also applied to remove disagreeable odours and flavours of medicinal plants, for example, Herba sargassii (Hai zao) is processed by a clear water rinse. Most herbs are sliced, shaved, or chopped, which is favourable for preparation, storage and pharmaceutical production.

The processing mechanism of Paozhi can be explained by a direct reduction of toxic contents and constituents, structural transformation of constituents and influence of excipients. Most Chinese Herbal Medicines (CHMs) need to be processed prior to use in clinical therapy. In the Chinese Pharmacopoeia, decoction pieces and related processing methods are laid out in specific chapters of CHM, and some decoction pieces are recorded with specific quality control standards and indications, such as Radix Astragali membranacei (Huang qi), which helps strengthening the immune response.

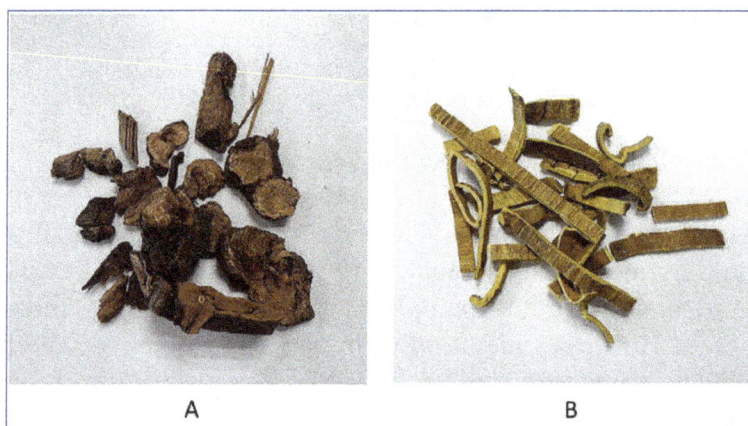

Paozhi processed root and bark samples. (A) Radix sanguisorba officinalis L. (Di yu). (B) Phellodendron chinese Schneid (Huang bai).

The earliest description of Paozhi can be traced back to 200 BC and classic methods, including burning, stewing and soaking with wine and vinegar, were recorded in 'Wu-Shi-Er-Bing-Fang'. In the Ming Dynasty (1368–1644 AD), the processing methods according to Paozhi flourished and became more refined and creative as a variety of additional excipients was introduced in herbal medicine processing. Later, in the first monograph of processing methods 'Lei-Gong-Pao-Zhi-Lun' (around the fifth century), the Paozhi processing methods of 268 TCM materials were recorded, of these, 178 medicines were prepared with excipients. These comply with the theory of 'seven-relation compatibility' in the TCM theory system. When two or more herbal TCMs are combined in one formula, the 'seven-relation compatibility' is applied, which is very important for Paozhi. For example, 'xiang wei' means one herbal medicine can reduce the toxicity of another medicine, thus the toxic herbal medicine *Rhizoma arisaematis Preparatum* (Tian nan xing) is traditionally processed with ginger to reduce its toxicity for clinical safety. Studies of chemical changes in processed Tian nan xing showed that levels of calcium oxalate, which is recognised as a toxic substance, were reduced by 50% compared to the raw herbal material. In 1662, processing methods of 439 Chinese medicines were described in the materia medica 'Pao-Zhi-Da-Fa'. In the Qing dynasty, the monograph of Paozhi method was recorded in the book 'Xin-Shi-Zhi-Nan', which encompassed many classic methods from the long history of processing herbal medicines.

Table: Commonly used Paozhi methods with examples of medicines.

Paozhi method	English translation	Excipient added	Examples of processed medicine
"Chao"	Stir-Frying	-	"Chao" Crataegi Fructus (Shan Zha)"
"Zhi"	Stir-Frying With Liquid Excipients	Yellow-Rice Wine	"Zhi" Radix Et Rhizome Rehi (Da Huang)
"Zheng"	Steaming	Vinegar	"Zheng" Schisandrae Chinensis Fructus (Wu Wei Zi)

Processing is the way that natural medicines are transformed into TCM by physical or chemical methods. Processing also increases efficacy and reduces inherent toxicity. The main processing methods encompass a variety of techniques such as cleaning, cutting, crushing, roasting, boiling, baking and stir-frying, with or without liquid/solid excipients. 'Chao' means stir-frying in Chinese. Clean and cut materials are stir-fried until a colour change to yellow is observed, or they may be either charred or 'carbonised'. Carbonised in 'chao' refers to decoction pieces that are black on the outside and brown on the inside. These three stages of processing represent a different degree of 'Chao' and infer a different medical efficacy. For example, *Crataegi fructus* (Shan zha) is used for enhancing digestion, which can be stir-fried into these three stages. Yellow 'Chao' Shan zha is usually used to treat indigestion and charred 'Chao'

Shan zha is used for diarrhoea, whereas, carbonised 'Chao' Shan zha is used for gastrointestinal haemorrhage.

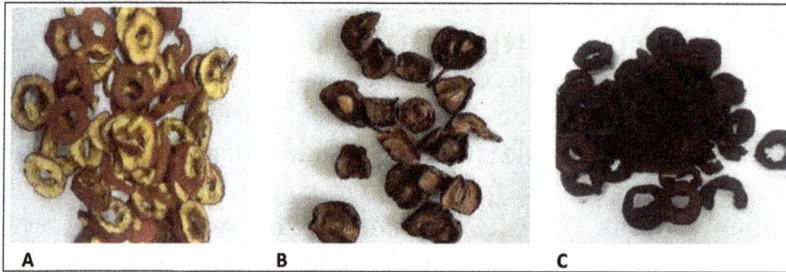

Three different methods of Paozhi processing of fruit slices (decoction pieces) of Crataegi Fructus (Shan zha): (A) Yellow 'Chao' (stir-fried until a colour change to yellow is observed). (B) Charred 'Chao' (stir-fried until a colour change to brown in achieved). (C) Carbonised 'Chao' (stir-fried until colour change to black on the outside and brown on the inside is attained).

'Zhi' means stir-frying with liquid excipients. Clean and cut material is stir-fried with a liquid, such as vinegar, salty water, honey, yellow rice wine or ginger sauce, which allows the liquid to be absorbed by the medical material. For instance, Radix Angelicae sinensis (Dang gui) is well-known to invigorate blood circulation in the human body, and this effect is enhanced when Dang gui is stir-fried with yellow rice wine. The chemical analysis of processed Radix Angelicae sinensis shows significant variation of the amount of ferulic acid and Z-ligustilide, and these chemicals are proved to have an effect in anti-platelet aggregation.

'Zheng' means steaming, which can alter the properties of a variety of herbal medicines. For instance, Radix polygoni Multiflora (He shou wu) is soaked with black bean sauce and then steamed in a non-ferrous container until the colour is changed into brown, then it is sliced into pieces and dried in the sun. The raw He shou wu is used for its anti-malarial properties, while 'Zhi' He shou wu has different therapeutic indications including improving the kidney function, hair blackening and strengthening of bones. Pharmacokinetic studies of typical constituents from processed Radix polygoni Multiflora by LC-ESI-MS/MS indicate that the processing method can improve the bioavailability of garlic acid and decrease the absorption of 2,3,5,4'-tetrahydroxystilbene-2-O-β-d-glucoside (PM-SG), resveratrol and emodin in rat plasma.

The different processing methods have varying influences on medicinal herbs, and this contributes to diverse medical activities and reduced toxicity. For example, *Radix et Rhizoma rhei* (Da huang) is commonly processed by four classical methods which are recorded in the Chinese Pharmacopoeia (2015). This encompasses 'Sheng' Da huang (dried raw material), 'Zhi' Da huang (stir-frying with wine), 'Zheng' Da huang (steaming with wine) and carbonised 'Chao' Da huang (stir-frying till carbonised). Each of these four processed Da huang products has different medical effects. 'Sheng' Da huang is often used for constipation in clinical practice, and 'Zhi' Da huang is effective for hematemesis, headache and toothache. Chemically, this may be explained by decomposition of conjugated anthraquinones into the corresponding free anthraquinones. 'Zhi' Da huang has an effect on constipation; however, the effect is weaker than for 'Sheng' Da huang, which enhances blood circulation, and this may result from decreased contents of tannins. Carbonised 'Chao' Da huang has an effect on haemostasis for hematochezia and no effect on blood circulation.

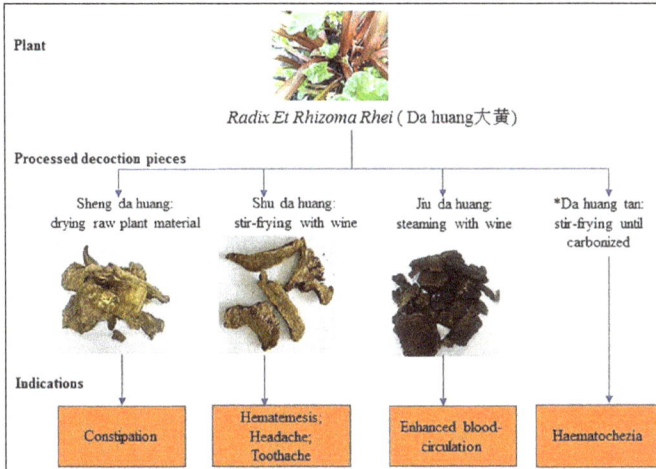

Examples of Da huang processed by different methods and applied for different indications. Da huang tan is rarely used, so an image is unavailable.

Nowadays, the difference between processed and non-processed medicines is studied by modern scientific analytic methods. For example, Radix aconiti (Chuan wu) is an essential herbal medicine, which has a long history of application in TCM as it has a wide range of medical effects, such as anti-inflammatory and analgesic properties. However, the non-processed Chuan wu is very toxic and induces remarkable neuro- and cardiotoxicity. Chuan wu is processed by boiling and drying. The comprehensive metabolomic characteristics of non-processed and processed samples were investigated by a LC-MS method, which identified specific metabolite changes. Diester diterpene alkaloids (DDA) and toxic monoester diterpene alkaloids (MDA) were identified to be the main components which were reduced by this processing method for Chuan wu. The contents of magnolo and honokiol from Cortex magnoliae Officinalis (Hou pu) were reduced by 14 and 40%, respectively, after processing by stir-frying with ginger, and the new component gingerol was formed. The solubility of active constituents can be improved to enhance the efficacy by processing, for instance, Huang lian, traditionally used for toothache, liver disease or inflammation and can be processed by stir-frying with wine, vinegar, salt, bile, or Fructus evodiae (Wu zhu yu). Chemical analysis of processed Huang lian suggests that the contents of alkaloids are different, depending on the processing method but all are higher than non-processed material, and stir-frying with wine leads to the highest contents.

Triterpene saponins were found to be the main bioactive constituents of Ginseng, which has anti-oxidant, anti-diabetic, immunomodulatory, anti-inflammatory and anti-cancer activities. After processing by steaming and drying, the chemical profiles are remarkably different between processed and non-processed Ginseng. The structural transformation of ginsenosides in processed Ginseng, which proved to have more potent bioactivities, contributes to its enhanced efficacy. Solubility is influenced by processing, and by the addition of excipients, such as wine, honey, vinegar, salt water and ginger juice. Excipients may react with constituents in herbal medicines and may have effects on active constituents, for example, it was reported that ginger juice has anti-inflammatory activity itself which contributes to the detoxification effect of processed *Rhizoma pinelliae Tematae* (Ban xia). Therefore, processing can result in reducing amounts of toxic constituents, structural transformation and solubility improvement of active constituents.

In addition to daodi, Paozhi also plays an important role in TCM in influencing the quality, safety and efficacy of medical materials. There is a continuing need for multidisciplinary research to fully evaluate the effects of these practices, in order to increase the understanding of their impact on the chemical fingerprints of therapeutic decoctions and on the mechanism of action of resultant TCMs. In different regions of China, the processing methods of TCM vary; for instance, white rice wine is commonly used in the Hunan province, but yellow rice wine is used in Fujian, Anhui and Guangxi province. Today, there is still no consistency of processing practice across China. Hong Kong is the international centre of TCM, and most of the TCM decoction pieces in the western world are imported from Hong Kong. It is reported that 66% of 365 kinds of TCM decoction pieces of commonly used TCM are processed locally in Hong Kong, where the processing methods are different to those in the mainland of China. Such differences may result in a Butterfly effect as eluded by Sheridan et al. and may result in very different therapeutic effects associated with the final TCM. Consistent and standardised processing methods are required for the global development of TCM.

In recent years, the study of Paozhi is focused on understanding and validating the traditional aspect of processing. The chemical profiles of processed herbal medicine are investigated by NMR, GC and LC-MS analysis methods, and metabolomic profiles are studied with chemical markers. In addition, toxicity or side-effects can result from improper processing methods, and therefore, a standardisation of processing methods for TCM is essential. It seems appropriate that in the modernisation of TCM, significant chemical contents and pharmacological indications should be applied as evaluation markers, a quality control standard should be established to reinforce the GMP of processed products, to optimise the process procedure and standardise the quality, safety and efficacy of decoction pieces.

Seven-relation Compatibility

Multiple herbs can be combined in TCM, with up to 20 herbs in one formula, yielding very complex decoctions. Such a complex formula is called Fangji in Chinese, and it is adjusted for each individual patient under the guidance of TCM theory. At times, single herbs are used to prepare decoctions for treatment, and for instance, *Radix Astragali membranacei* (Huang qi) is used on its own to treat lung disease. The combination of herbs within one formula is under the guidance of the 'seven-relation compatibility', which includes the following: 'mutual accentuation', 'mutual enhancement', 'mutual counteraction', 'mutual suppression', 'mutual antagonism' and 'mutual incompatibility' between two herbs. In addition, single herbs can be used under the 'seven-relation compatibility' in an 'individual application' for the treatment of certain diseases.

Table: Explanation and application of 'seven-relation compatibility'.

Chinese name	English Translation	Explanation	Example of Application
Xiang xu	"Mutual accentuation"	Two medicinal herbs which have similar effects are applied together to achieve better efficacy.	Ginseng Is Combined With Radix Astragali Membranacei To Improve The "Qi" And The Therapeutic Efficacy.
Xiang shi	"Mutual enhancement"	Two medicinal herbs which have different effects but can be combined to enhance the effect of the main medicinal herb.	Poria Cocos Wolf Is Applied With Huang Qi To Improve The Efficacy Of Huang Qi.
Xiang wei	"Mutual counteraction"	Two medicinal herbs applied together because one of them can reduce the toxicity of the another.	Ginger Can Reduce The Neurotoxicity Of Rhizome Pinelliae Tematae's.
Xiang sha	"Mutual suppression"	Two medicinal herbs are applied together because one of them can eliminate the toxicity of the another one.	Ginger Can Suppress Numbing And Paralytic Effects On The Respiratory System Of Rhizome Arisaematis Preparatum.
Xiang wu	"Mutual antagonism"	The therapeutic effects will be eliminated if the two medicinal herbs are applied together.	Semen Raphani Decreases Ginseng's Efficacy.
Xiang fan	"Mutual incompatibility"	Two herbs which can be safely used separately will exert toxicity if they are applied together.	When Wu Tou Applied With Rhizome Pinelliae Tematae They Exert Toxicity In The CNS System.
Dan Xing	"Individual application"	One medicinal herb can be applied on its own.	Radix Astragali Membranacei Is Used To Treat Lung Disease.

Fangji

Fangji is defined as formulae composed of multiple herbs with integrated medical effects, and it is guided by 'Jun Chen Zuo Shi' theory. One TCM formula generally consists of four different kinds of herbal medicine, which is called 'jun', 'chen', 'zuo' and 'shi'. Each of them plays a different role within the formula. All of these medicinal herbs work harmoniously together to achieve therapeutic effects and bring the balance of Yin and Yang back to the human body. In the TCM formula theory system, 'jun' means the 'master' and provides the principal therapeutic effect for the disease; and 'chen' represents the 'advisor' which functions as the second principal medicinal component, supporting the medical efficacy of the 'jun' medicine. 'Zuo' represents the 'soldier' and is applied to treat associated symptoms or reduce toxicity of the 'jun' medicine. 'Shi' represents the 'guide' which can direct other medicines to the diseased organ or contribute to the harmony of all herbs in the formula. For instance, *Radix glycyrrhizae* (Gan cao) is the most commonly used 'shi' medicine, since its sweet flavour can improve the taste of formula decoction and enhance the harmony of the combined herbs. For single-herb formulas, the medicinal herb is a 'jun' medicine (master medicine), which shows the principal medical effects.

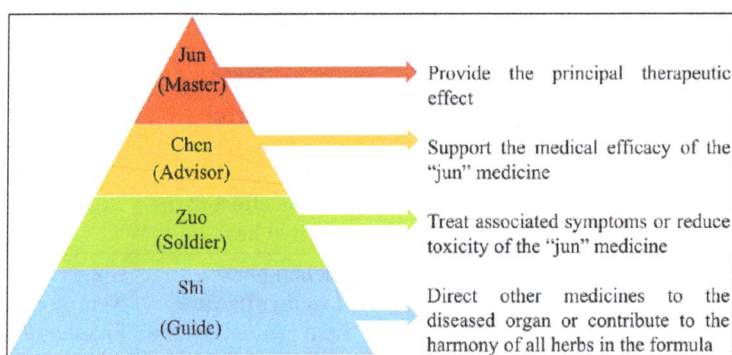

The principle of 'Jun Chen Zuo Shi' theory.

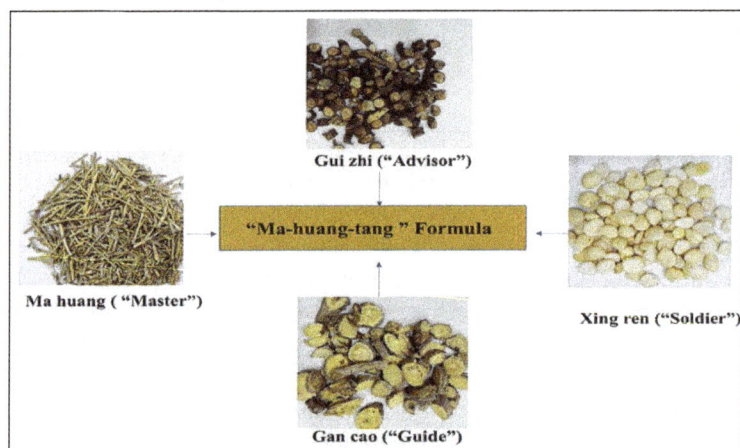

Composition of herbs and roles in 'Ma-huang-tang' formula.

For example, 'Ma-huang-tang' is a formula traditionally used to treat inflammatory liver disease and consists of *Ephedra sinica* Stapf (Ma huang), *Ramulus cinnamomi Cassiae* (Gui zhi), *Semen pruni Armeniacae* (Xing ren) and *Radix glycyrrhizae* (Gan cao). Ma huang works as the master medicine, which provides the main anti-inflammatory effects in the treatment of lung diseases. Gui zhi works as the advisor medicine and assists Ma huang to function well, which compiles the 'xiang shi' ('mutual enhancement') from the 'seven-relation compatibility'. Xing ren is the soldier medicine and enhances the efficacy of Ma huang. Gan cao functions as the guide medicine, which can adjust the properties of other medicines and improve the harmonisation in the formula. The overall efficacy of the TCM formula is a result of the mixture of chemical components in the multiple medicinal herbs. However, it was reported that pure and active components which were separated and purified from single or multiple herbs are different in their chemical profile when compared to traditional decoctions. This may be due to synergistic effects in the complex medicine or to chemical reactions and other changes which may occur during the decoction procedure.

Formulations of TCM

Decoctions

Decoction is the earliest and most commonly used preparation method in the clinical application of TCM. A TCM decoction is the herbal tea that is made of processed medicinal herbs which are simmered for hours. The preparation of a traditional medicine decoction has multiple steps such as the sequence of boiling the herbal material and different boiling and filtering times. The preparation of a decoction is complex, as it requires experience and often takes considerable time. The herbal ingredients within the formula for decoction can be changed for the individual patient according to the disease. The herbal medicine may include leaves, flowers, roots, bark or fruits, and the procedure of preparation is depending on the part of the herb that is used. It is of concern that in some instances, the quality and stability of herbal material cannot be assured. Also, the unpleasant flavour of a decoction has been a problem for patients for thousands of years. As equipment advances and market demand increases, modern decoctions have become very popular in TCM hospitals, because of convenience. Decoctions have a quick and often complete absorption with good bioavailability. In a modernised decoction method, the medicinal herbs are combined with water and are extracted in TCM decoction machines. Modern formulations also include granules, oral liquids, tablets, capsules and injections. This change in methodology may in fact influence the composition of the final TCM, and this is another area that would benefit from comparative research studies directed at classical and modern decoction methods.

Modern Granular Formulations

The use of granules has dramatically increased in China since they are easy to handle, store and formulate. The granule made of a single herb is called a single dispensing granule; when made of multiple herbs, it is called a dispensing formula granule. The preparation of granules is included in the extensive process of decoction: they are prepared by decoction or aqueous extraction with the aid of suitable excipients. After being dissolved in warm water, they can be ingested by patients. With the increasing development of TCM granules, international research has focused on whether decoction can be replaced by granules with similar effectiveness and safety. During the procedure of granule preparation, the difference of water extraction, concentration, desiccation and granulation may influence the dissolution and chemical profiles of active ingredients. Thus, this may result in different clinical efficacy between granules and decoction.

Recently, some cases related to the equivalence of effect between granules and decoction have been reported. Indeed, some differences in chemical consistency were identified, which suggest that the efficacy might not be equivalent between both forms of medicine. Ge-Gen-Qin-Lian-Tang is a classic TCM formula for the treatment of inflammatory bowel disease. The comparison of chemical fingerprints of traditional decoction and granules of Ge-Gen-Qin-Lian-Tang was investigated by liquid chromatography-diode array detector (LC-DAD) to ensure the consistency of efficacy. The fingerprints demonstrated small variations among the 20 peaks, but the peak area of puerain, berberine and baicalein from the granule sample was 50% less than that of the decoction. The TCM formula Da-Cheng-Qi-Tang is commonly used to treat digestive disease. The chemical consistency of decoctions of Da-Cheng-Qi-Tang prepared by traditional and modern methods was investigated. Five compounds were identified as chemical markers, an analysis of which established that the chemical fingerprints were not consistent between these two kinds of decoctions. The study showed that the traditional decoction method had a stronger purgative effect due to higher concentrations of rhein and sennosides. Therefore, it is very important to understand the impact of the formulation method on the therapeutic effect of a final granular TCM product.

Fingerprint-efficacy Analysis in TCM

Over the past 30 years, chromatographic and spectrophotometric fingerprinting methods have dramatically improved, and the application of hyphenated techniques such as high performance liquid chromatography (HPLC)-mass spectrometry (HPLC-MS), liquid chromatography-nuclear magnetic resonance (LC-NMR) or gas chromatography mass spectrometry (GC-MS) in the analysis of TCM facilitates the determination of the quality in research and in the pharmaceutical industry. However, quality standards are challenging to establish, because the complexity of potential active ingredients in medicinal herbs is used in TCM. Today, commonly applied models for TCM quality control include conventional methods, such as microscopic, and macroscopic identification and comparison with monographs, chemical fingerprint analysis using thin-layer liquid chromatography (TLC), liquid chromatography (LC), HPLC, gas chromatography (GC), GC-MS, etc. and multiple marker assays.

Chemical fingerprints and bioactivities assay linked with multiple markers is currently recognised to be effective for TCM analysis. The use of known and previously characterised markers for the analysis of constituents is the most popular method for identification and quality control in TCM. For example, the ginsenoside fingerprint profiles are applied for the authentication of Panax species. The spectrum of ultra-performance liquid chromatography tandem mass spectrometry (UPLC-MS/MS) of three batches of Goji was correlated with the biological data using 2,2-diphenyl-1-picrylhydrazyl (DPPH) and 2,2'-azino-bis(3-ethylbenzothiazoline-6-sulphonic acid) (ABTS) assays. Compounds relating to the antioxidant activity of Goji, such as chlorogenic acid, quercetin and kaempferol, were subsequently identified by analysis of UPLC-MS/MS data.

Because of TCM's complexity, it is rare that any single ingredient provides the overall evidence for medical efficacy. Chemometric methods, such as similarity evaluation or principal component analysis, are often used to investigate the fingerprint and bioactivity relationship within the TCM. GC-MS is usually applied for the analysis of volatile metabolites, whereas LC-MS is often used to identify and quantify non-volatile components. Hyphenated methods, such as LC-MS can provide information on fragments of constituents, which can help in the elucidation and identification of chemical structures. In recent years, LC-MS analysis has been widely used in TCM due to its high sensitivity, selectivity and generation of specific information. NMR metabolomic profiling is currently recognised as a quick and generic method in the study and quality control of TCM material. For instance, it was reported that the quality control of *Radix Angelica Sinensis* was studied by NMR profiling, which resulted in observed differences between samples prepared by different methods.

To ensure the consistency of herbal medicine, the concept of phyto-equivalence was developed. Phyto-equivalence is a comparison of the chromatographic fingerprint of a herbal medicine with the profile of a standard reference product. The fingerprint is defined as a characteristic profile, which reflects the overall complex chemical composition of the sample analysed by chromatographic or electrophoretic techniques. Chromatographic fingerprints are accepted by the US Food and Drug Administration (FDA) in applications for new product approvals. In TCM studies, fingerprints could provide a complete set of information of chemical components including the relative quantity of all detectable analytes. Fingerprinting is widely used to authenticate or differentiate between species, geographical regions or processing methods in TCM.

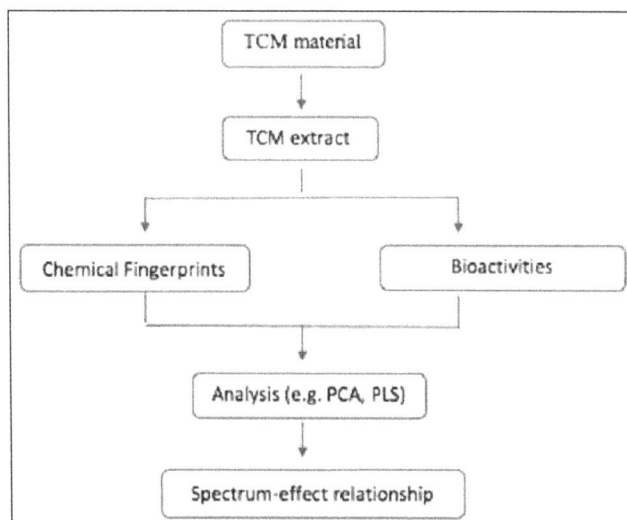

The method of 'fingerprint-efficacy relationship' in TCM.

The 'fingerprint-efficacy relationship' is a method that associates TCM fingerprints with a specific pharmacological effect. Multiple methods relate chemical fingerprints, such as characteristic peaks, to bioactivities. The 'fingerprint-efficacy relationship' investigation procedure involves finding the appropriate analytical methods for fingerprints, identifying assays for the various bioactivities, using statistical methods to find the fingerprint-efficacy relationship, select candidate components, and validation of the bioactivities of the identified candidate components. For instance, Valeriana jatamansi Jones (Zhi zhu xiangI) has a long history of use in TCM to treat mood disorders like anxiety. The 'fingerprint-efficacy relationship' was studied by correlating HPLC fingerprints with in vitro and in vivo tests. Four chemical components, hesperidin, isochlorogenic acid A, isochlorogenic B and isochlorogenic C are regarded as multiple biological markers for this anti-anxiety effect.

Principal component analysis (PCA) is a statistical method, which can reduce the number of variables and dimensionality and create principal components (PCs) to explain the variables in original data. PCA is usually combined with cluster analysis, correlation analysis or regression analysis to determine the relationship of fingerprints and efficacy. It extracts data and can remove redundant information to focus on the main factors. PCA is often used together with other chemometric methods due to the lack of a specific quantification mathematical model for variables. For example, *Andrographis herba* (Chuan xin lian) is well-known in China because of its bitter taste, which is one of the five flavours in TCM theory. The bitter flavour is recognised as relating to the pharmacological effects of *Andrographis herba*. In Zhang's group, the chemical components of 30 different types of *Andrographis herba* and fingerprint spectrum were determined by HPLC, and the PCA was applied to analyse the chemical components relating to bitter taste relating. According to the results from PCA, andrographolide, neoandrographolide, 1,4-deoxyandrographolide and dehyandrographhlide were determined as substances responsible for the bitter flavour of Chuan xin lian. *Ephedra sinica* Stapf (Ma huang) is commonly applied for rheumatism, asthma, fever and rheumatoid arthritis in China. The significance of the inorganic elements of Ma huang from different geographical regions was studied by using elemental plasma mass spectroscopy fingerprints and PCA, and the study showed that this is an effective strategy to discriminate TCM samples.

Basic Theories of Traditional Chinese Medicine

TCM theory in its present form arose from the naturalistic philosophies of ancient China, influenced and expanded upon by the accumulated clinical experience of generations of literate scholar practitioners. It is because of this cultural context that TCM theory can at times seem abstruse or outdated. However, it represents a complete, integrated method of interpreting human physiology and responding to pathological changes in the body.

The most important concepts taken from ancient Chinese naturalistic philosophy in TCM are those of qi, yinyang, and the five phases (wuxing). Theoretical concepts specific to TCM include the doctrine of zheng ti guang nian, the concepts of the viscera and bowels (zangfu xue shuo), channels and networks (jingluo), body sub- stances (qi, blood, essence and body fluids qi xue jing jinye); and pathogenic agents (bing yin). These theories, together with the methodologies of the four (diagnostic) methods (si zhen) and pattern discrimination (bian zheng) comprise the theoretical framework of TCM. Each of the therapeutic tools of TCM, including acupuncture and moxibustion (zhenjiu), Chinese herbology (zhongyao fang), and Chinese thera- peutic massage (zhongyi tuina) rest upon this theoretical basis.

Yinyang Theory (Yinyang Xue Shuo)

Yinyang theory expresses a universal standard of quality that describes two complemen- tary, opposite aspects of an indivisible whole. It is used to describe function and relationship of these aspects as part of a continuous process of transformation and change in the universe. Applied to medicine, yinyang theory is used to compare and contrast, and thus differentiate, physiological and pathological phenomena.

Yin is associated to qualities such as cold, rest, responsiveness, passivity, darkness, structure, the interior, downward and inward motion, and decrease. By contrast, yang is associated with heat, stimulation, movement, activity, light, the exterior, upward and outward motion, and increase. It is important to observe that these aspects occur only in relation to each other (i.e., cold can be defined only by the knowledge of heat, darkness by the presence or absence of light, and so on). In medicine, yinyang theory would be applied to opposites such as structure (yin) and function (yang), the lower body (yin) in relation to the upper body (yang); however, the concepts of yinyang are never absolute. They are applied to given objects in order to express their relation to other objects, actions, or processes.

Yinyang theory has four fundamental characteristics, known as the four relations of yinyang:

- Opposition,

- Interdependence, interdivisibility, and relativity,

- Inter-consuming-supporting,

- Intertransforming.

Opposition

Yinyang theory describes a universal qualitative standard. One of the key aspects of this is that the yin aspect of something exists only in op- position to its yang aspect. Heaven and earth, sun and moon, night and day, male and female, up and down, inside and outside, and quiescence and movement are manifestations of a duality intrinsic to the universe. Water is cold and fire is hot, and water flows downward while fire tends to rise. Therefore, water is yin and fire is yang. Similarly, day is yang and night is yin, high is yang and low is yin, matter is yin and energy is yang, and the passive element is yin and the active element is yang.

In terms of medicine, the upper body is yang in relation to the lower body, which is yin. However, the anterior side of the body is yin while the posterior side is yang. The medial aspect of the extremities is yin while the lateral aspect is yang. As a whole, the interior of the body is yin while the exterior is yang. Within the inte- rior of the body, the zang organs (sometimes called "viscera"), considered "solid" and in charge of storage, are yin, whereas the fu organs (sometimes referred to as "bowels") are held to be "hollow" and in charge of discharging their contents, and thus are yang. Diseases that manifest signs and symptoms associated with heat and excessive metabolic activity are yang, whereas diseases that display cold signs and a decrease in activity are yin. Rapid, replete, forceful pulses are yang, whereas slow, vacuous, and forceless are yin. Medicinal substances are classified as hot or warm (yang) and cool or cold (yin). Overall yin refers to structure and form in the body, as opposed to function and metabolic activity, which are yang.

Table: Basic yinyang correspondences used in TCM.

Yin	Yang
Water	Fire
Cold	Hot
Interior	Exterior
Slow	Rapid
Passivity	Activity
Quiescence	Movement
Lower position or downward direction	Upper position or upward direction
Interior position or inward direction	Exterior position or outward direction
Dimness	Brightness
Inhibition	Excitation
Weakness	Strength
Hypoactivity	Hyperactivity
Structure	Function
Internal organs	Body surface
Zang organs	Fu organs
Lower body, below the waist	Upper body, above the waist
Anterior region	Posterior region
Medial aspect of the limbs	Lateral aspect of the limbs
Right side	Left side
Qi	Blood

Interdependence

Yin and yang define aspects of a whole, and therefore, they depend on each other. The whole is defined by the existence of the two opposing aspects. "Cold" cannot be defined without "heat," "above" is meaningless without "below," and "exterior" and "interior" mutually define each other. This is all in relation to a whole that contains these two parts.

In medicine, the clearest example of yinyang interdependence is the relationship between structure and function. Structure (or form) pertains to yin, and function to yang. Together, they are complementary aspects of the whole that is the living body. Sufficient substance (structure) in the form of body fluids, healthy tissue, etc., allows for normal function. In turn, only when the functional processes are in good condition can the essential substances be appropriately replenished. The balance between structure and function is the basis for healthy physiological activity.

Interdivisibility and Relativity: Because yinyang are aspects of the whole, no object, phenomenon, event, or situation can ever be labeled as purely or wholly yin or yang. Phenomena in the universe have yin and yang aspects, depending on the viewpoint of analysis. For example, day is considered yang when compared with night, but the early hours of the day (before noon) are yang when compared with the hours after noon, which are yin. In Chinese thought, it is said that the morning is yang within yang, and the afternoon is yin within yang. These hierarchies of yin and yang can be extended ad infinitum, as each separate phenomenon can be divided into its yin and yang aspect.

Inter-consuming-supporting

In yinyang theory, a gain, growth, or advance of one aspect of the whole means a loss, decline, or retreat of the other (this is sometimes referred to as "the waxing and waning" of yin and yang). Under normal conditions, this consumption/support occurs within limits. In terms of physiology, it could be likened to homeostasis. Exceeding these limits results in dysfunction and disease, but here too, we may see the consumption of one by the other. A yang disorder, with an excess of metabolic activity, will gradually consume the resources (yin) of the body. Conversely, cold congelation or advanced age (yin) can bring about a drastic reduction of body function (yang). In terms of pathology, all diseases can be thought of as pertaining to one of four imbalances along these lines: excess of yang, excess of yin, deficiency of yang, or deficiency of yin.

Intertransformation

This back and forth between yin and yang implies a characteristic of constant motion and transformation, which is observed in the world. Yin transforms into yang, and yang in turn evolves into yin. The yang day transforms into the yin night, just like shadows moving across the face of a mountain as the sun travels across the horizon.

In terms of medicine, the intertransformation of yinyang can be said to occur in two ways: harmoniously, as in the natural course of development, growth, aging, and death, and deviating from the norm, as in response to drastic environmental changes or internal imbalance. Normally, yin and yang follow each other naturally, and this constant transformation is the source of life as we observe it. We could call this smooth, successive process as "health." In disease, this process is disrupted and yin and yang are out of balance—an excess of one, which automatically pre-supposes a deficiency of the other. This can continue to the point where inter-transformation occurs, but as a progression of disease. Chinese medical thought holds that "when the exuberance of yin reaches and extreme, it will transform into yang; when heat blazes, it transforms into cold." This is observable when, for example, a very high fever (which would be a yang disorder) causes shock with hypothermia, loss of consciousness, etc. (yin symptoms).

Application in Traditional Chinese Medicine

Yinyang theory permeates every aspect of TCM. As can be seen from the examples, it is used as a framework to understand anatomy, physiology, pathology, diagnosis, and treatment. Its importance cannot be overrated.

Five-phase (Wuxing) Theory

Five-phase theory establishes a system of correspondences that groups phenomena in the universe into five categories. These categories represent tendencies of movement and transformation in the universe, and are associated with the natural phenomena of wood (mu), fire (huo), earth (tu), metal (jin), and water (shui). Clear, constant relationships between them are used to explain changes in nature.

Five-phase Categorization

Each of the phases represents a category of related functions and qualities. Wood is associated with the season of spring, sprouting, early growth, awakening, morning, childhood, and the penetrating, powerful impetus of new life, anger, and wind. Fire is associated with summer. It represents a maximum state of activity, flourishing, exuberant growth, outward motion, high noon, and the expansive movement of happiness and open flame. Earth is associated with the long summer (or the transition between seasons). It signals balance and equilibrium, the early afternoon, nourishment, abundance, the quiet of pensiveness and worry, and dampness. Metal is associated with the autumn season, declining function, a movement toward crystallization and shedding that is not needed, dusk, clarity and sadness, and dry weather. Water is associated with winter. It expresses a state of downward motion, accumulation, rest, nighttime, and the development of new potential, the concentration of willpower and fear, and the cold.

Five phase correspondences permeate all aspects of classical thought in China. The five-way categorization is applied to colors, sounds, odors, flavors, emotions, animals, the planets, and ultimately everything in the universe.

Relationships between the Five Phases

The five phases succeed each other in cycles, acting upon each other in fixed ways. Two cyclical relationships are held to exist among the five phases: an engendering (sheng) cycle and a controlling (ke) cycle. Both of these cycles are deemed to be natural and necessary. Without engenderment, there is no life; without control, things become excessive.

Table: Five-phase correspondences.

	Wood	Fire	Earth	Metal	Water
Direction	East	South	Center	West	North
Season	Spring	Summer	Late summer	Fall	Winter
Climate	Wind	Heat	Dampness	Dryness	Cold
Planet	Jupiter	Mars	Saturn	Venus	Mercury
Number	3+5=8	2+5=7	5	4+5=9	1+5=6
Meat	Chicken	Goat	Beef	Horse	Pork
Cereal	Wheat	Millet	Sorghum	Rice	Beans (soy)
Sound	Jiao	Zheng	Gong	Shang	Yu
Musical note	C	D	E	G	A
Color	Green	Red	Yellow	White	Black
Taste	Bitter	Acid	Sweet	Pungent	Salt
Smell	Uremic	Burnt	Scented	Cool	Putrid
Organ	Liver	Heart	Spleen	Lung	Kidney
Viscera	Urinary bladder	Small intestine	Stomach	Large intestine	Bladder
Senses organ	Eyes	Tongue	Mouth	Nose	Ear
Tissue	Tendons	Vessels	Muscles	Skin	Bones
Bodily sounds	Hu (sigh)	Laugh	Singing	Crying	Moan
Virtues	Benevolence	Courtesy	Fidelity	Justice	Knowledge
Emotion	Anger	Joy	Worry	Melancholy	Fear
Spiritual activity	Hun	Shen	Yi	Po	Zhi
Bodily region	Neck, nape	Thoracocostal	Spine	Escapulodorsal	Lumbar

Engendering Cycle: This is the cycle whereby the phases are believed to proceed in order to generate each other in an orderly sequence. The natural action or movement of one phase fosters the growth or waxing of the next, thus wood engenders fire, fire engenders earth, earth engenders metal, metal engenders water, and water engenders wood. This cycle is also known as the "Mother-Son" relationship, with the engendering phase acting as "mother" to the next (the "son").

Controlling Cycle: This cycle follows the sequence in which the phases suppress, control, or inhibit each other. In this sequence, wood controls earth, earth controls water, water controls fire, fire controls metal, and metal controls wood.

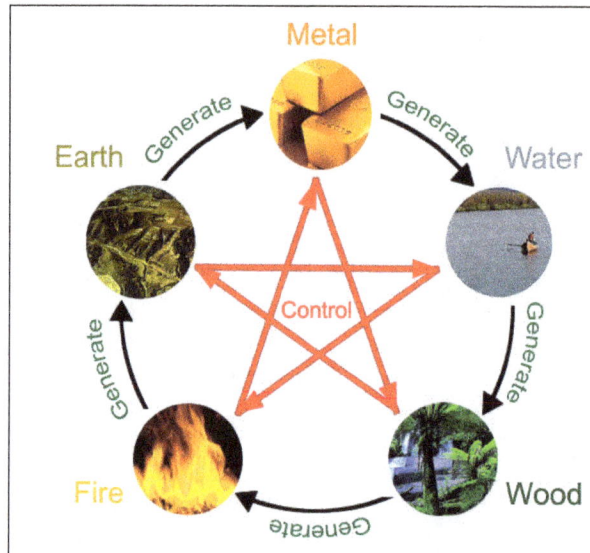

The five phases (engendering and controlling cycles.

Thus, all phases stand in relationship to the others in one of the four ways: engendering, being engendered, controlling, and being controlled. It follows that the state of one phase in the system is always dependent on the condition of the others. If viewed as aspects of an organic whole, the actions of control and engenderment exerted by each of the phases add up to maintain a dynamic balance.

Five-phase Theory in Traditional Chinese Medicine

Five-phase correspondences exist in TCM as well. The viscera (zang) and bowels (fu), along with the acupuncture channels, are classified in this system. Five-phase theory is also used to interpret the physiology and pathology of the human body in relation to the natural environment. It is likewise applied to etiology, diagnosis, treatment, and prognosis.

The main five-phase correspondences used in TCM are those of the zang organs: wood is attributed to the liver, which regulates free flow of qi; fire is attributed to the heart, which promotes the warming of the whole body; earth is attributed to the spleen, which is in charge of the transportation and transformation of food; metal is attributed to the lung, which promotes the descending of qi; and water is attributed to the kidney, which is responsible for the storage of essence and regulating body fluids. The basic engendering and controlling relationships of the five phases are interpreted as follows in physiology.

Engendering Cycle

- Wood engenders fire: The liver stores blood and supplements the blood to be regulated by the heart.

- Fire engenders earth: The heart provides warmth, which is indispensable for the spleen to function.

- Earth engenders metal: The spleen transforms and transports the essential nutrients and sends them up to replenish the lung and support its activity.

- Metal engenders water: The lung, with its clearing and descending functions, sends down yin fluids to the kidneys.

- Water engenders wood: Kidney essence nourishes liver blood.

Controlling Cycle

- Wood controls earth: The liver's dredging effect prevents spleen qi from becoming stagnant.

- Fire controls metal: The upward and outward movement of heart fire prevents lung qi from descending excessively.

- Earth controls water: The action of transportation of the spleen prevents the fluids controlled by the kidney from overflowing.

- Metal controls wood: The clearing and descending action of the lung counteracts the ascent of liver qi.

- Water controls fire: Kidney yin flows upward to nourish heart yin, thus restricting heart yang.

Five-phase Theory in Disease Causation

The engendering and controlling cycles of the five phases are used to explain disease causation, mainly through the "Mother-Son" relationship. In addition, a condition of excess or deficiency in one of the organs can affect other organs by altering the relationships of engenderment and control.

Disease Causation through the "Mother-Son" Relationship

- Disease of the Mother affecting the Son: If the Mother becomes deficient, it will be unable to nourish the Son, and will eventually cause a deficiency of the Son. For example, a deficiency of the kidney essence (water) will negatively impact the production of liver blood (wood), gradually inducing a condition of liver deficiency. Conversely, if the Mother is affected by an excess condition, this may cause the Son to become excessive as well. For example, if liver fire (wood) flares upward, it will cause heart fire (fire) to become exuberant, leading to an overabundance of fire in the liver and heart.

- Disease of the Son affecting the Mother: In most cases, a disease of the Son will induce a deficiency of the Mother. For example, a deficiency of kidney yin can induce a deficiency of lung yin, leading to deficiency of both organs. This is explained as due to the increased supply from the Mother to the deficient Son eventually exhausting the resources of the Mother.

Disease Causation through Deficiency or Excess of an Organ

- Deficiency of one of the organs can induce any of the following scenarios:

    ◦ Deficiency of the Son due to reduction of nourishment.

    ◦ Deficiency of the Mother due to increased demand for nourishment.

    ◦ Overcontrolling from its controller, which would aggravate the deficiency.

    ◦ Counter-domination by its controlled organ.

- Excess of one of the organs can result in any of the following:

    ◦ Excess of the Son.

    ◦ Excess of the Mother.

    ◦ Over-controlling of its controlled organ, causing debilitation of the latter.

    ◦ Counter-domination of its controlling organ, causing its debilitation.

Theory of the Viscera and Bowels (Zangfu)

Traditional Chinese medical theory describes physiology as a system of functional spheres of influence, known as the zangfu. Loosely correlated to the anatomical structures described by western biomedicine, the "organs" of Chinese medicine interact with one another, and with inputs from the exterior, in predictable, organized ways that constitute the normal activity of the system. Changes and deviations in zangfu function can be observed from exterior manifestations, which constitute patterns of disharmony, i.e., disease. At the core of the system are the five zang (viscera): lung, heart, liver, spleen, and kidney. All of the other tissues of the body, including sense organs, connective tissues, fluids, excretions, and the six fu (bowels: large intestine, small intestine, gallbladder, stomach, bladder, and the Sanjiao) are seen as subordinated to the zang, which thus represent entire systems of related function. These organ systems are at the core of TCM practice. Diagnosis and treatment all refer there and are ultimately directed toward one or more of the zangfu.

Table: The five transport-shu points of the yin channels.

	Jing-Well (wood)	Ying-Spring (fire)	Shu-Stream (earth)	Jing-River (metal)	He-Sea (water)
Liver (wood)	Dadun LR 1	Xingjian LR 2	Taichong LR 3	Zhongfeng LR 4	Ququan LR 8
Heart (fire)	Shaochong HT 9	Shaofu HT 8	Shenmen HT 7	Lingdao HT 4	Shaohai HT 3
Pericardium (fire)	Zhongchong PC 9	Laogong PC 8	Daling PC 7	Jianshi PC 5	Quze PC 3
Spleen (earth)	Yinbai SP 1	Dadu SP 2	Taibai SP 3	Shangqiu SP 5	Yinlingquan SP 9
Lung (metal)	Shaoshang LU 11	Yuji LU 10	Taiyuan LU 9	Jingqu LU 8	Chize LU 5
Kidney (water)	Yongquan KI 1	Rangu KI 2	Taixi KI 3	Fuliu KI 7	Yingu KI 10

Table: "Mother-Son" points of the 12 regular channels.

Channel	Mother point (for tonification)	Son point (for dispersion)
Liver (wood)	Ququan (LR 8) (water)	Xingjian (LR 2) (fire)
Heart (fire)	Shaochong (HT 9) (wood)	Shenmen (HT 7) (earth)
Pericardium (fire)	Zhongchong (PC 9) (wood)	Daling (PC 7) (earth)
Spleen (earth)	Dadu (SP 2) (fire)	Shangqiu (SP 5) (metal)
Lung (metal)	Taiyuan (LU 9) (earth)	Chize (LU 5) (water)
Kidney (water)	Fuliu (KI 7) (metal)	Yongquan (KI 1) (wood)
Gallbladder (wood)	Xiaxi (GB 43) (water)	Yangfu (GB 38) (fire)
Small Intestine (fire)	Houxi (SI 3) (wood)	Xiaohai (SI 8) (earth)
Sanjiao (fire)	Zhongzhu (SJ 3) (wood)	Tianjing (SJ 10) (earth)
Stomach (earth)	Jiexi (ST 41) (fire)	Lidui (ST 45) (metal)
Large Intestine (metal)	Quchi (LI 11) (earth)	Erjian (LI 2) (water)
Urinary Bladder (water)	Zhiyin (UB 67) (metal)	Shugu (UB 65) (wood)

Six Fu

In contrast with the zang, which are solid in structure and in charge of various functions of storage and construction, the fu are said to be hollow, and their functions relate to the passage of substances through the body (mostly food). An adage in TCM goes, "The five zang store but do not drain; the six fu drain but do not store." Proper function of the fu implies constant motion. Their pathology is frequently keyed to obstruction of the free passage by various pathogens.

Briefly, the six fu and their functions are as follows:

- The stomach (wei), considered the "chief" of the fu, is in charge of receiving the food we eat. Its function is called the "rotting and ripening" of food and pertains to the initial stages of digestion. It is associated with the spleen.

- The small intestine (xiao chang) is understood as being in charge of separat- ing "the clear from the turbid" along with the large intestine (da chang), which also oversees the formation and expulsion of stool. Although associated with the heart and the lung, respectively, their functions are more relevant to those of the spleen and stomach.

- The gallbladder (dan) stores bile and participates in the liver's coursing and discharging functions; in TCM, it is said to be associated with the capacity for resolve, decision-making, and taking action.

- The urinary bladder (pang guang) handles the expulsion of fluids managed by the kidney.

- The sanjiao is unique to TCM. It is known as "the fu with function but no form," it is believed to be the "triple furnace" where the functions of the rest of the zangfu take place. The organs are housed within the three chambers of the san- jiao (upper, middle, and lower). The sanjiao, along with the lung, spleen, and kidney, is also in charge of "the waterways" of the body, i.e., its function involves the transmission of fluids throughout the body.

Etiology and Pathophysiology in Traditional Chinese Medicine

As has been emphasized, TCM has a unique way of looking at health and illness. It does not rely on animistic or magical explanations for disease causation, yet it also does not recognize the existence of pathogens the way Western biomedicine does. From a TCM perspective, the virus or bacterium is not the causative agent per se, but one of the intermediate contributing factors for development of disease. Ac- cording to TCM theory, the fundamental factor in etiology is weakness of the body's normal function, referred to as zheng qi. Once zheng qi has been weakened for whatever reason (sudden weather changes, emotional upsets, overexertion, poor eating habits, and so on), particular conditions arise that manifest as dysfunction. Disease thus arises when the balance of the body's processes (structure and func- tion, qi and blood, zangfu, and the channel system) is lost. In lieu of this initial disharmony, says TCM theory, no disease can arise. The Neijing Suwen, the oldest extant text on TCM theory, says "Yin is calm, yang is hidden, therefore the spirit is at rest." This condition of balance extends to the relationship between the body and its surrounding environment. Quoting from the Suwen again, "Yinyang of the four seasons are the beginning and end of all things, the root of life and death. To go against them damages life; to follow their course prevents the arisal of disease." TCM thus classifies pathogenic factors according to their origin:

- Exogenous: Also known as "the six weather evils" (liu yin), these are wind (feng), cold (han), damp (shi), dryness (zao), summer heat (shu), and heat (re). Also classified in this category is pestilential qi (li qi), i.e., epidemic diseases.

- Endogenous: The "seven emotions" (qi qing) (anger, euphoria, worry, sadness, fear, melancholy, and fright) are said to adversely affect the flow of qi, thus giving rise to disharmony and disease.

- Miscellaneous: "Neither exogenous nor endogenous," this category includes all aspects of a disorderly lifestyle, such as poor diet, binging and starving, fatigue due to physical or mental overexertion, and excessive sexual activity. It also includes traumatic injury, parasites, poisonous bites, poisoning, and incorrect medical treatment. There are also the so-called "secondary pathogenic factors, such as blood stasis (xue yu) and phlegm (tan), which arise as the result of the others, but which in turn cause or complicate disease conditions.

Exogenous Pathogens: Six Evils (Liu Yin/Liu Xie)

The exogenous pathogens are those that attack the body from the exterior and in- clude the so called "six weather evils" and "pestilential qi." The ancient Chinese sages observed the effects of exposure on the human body, and determined that six climactic conditions could affect the yinyang balance of the organism. These six influences, namely wind, cold, damp, dryness, summer heat, and heat, adversely affect health when they change suddenly and surpass the body's capacity to adapt or when preexisting imbalance makes the body susceptible to their pathogenic effects. Put otherwise, these influences are part of nature. It is only when they occur abruptly or when the organism is already weakened that they become etiological factors.

Under certain circumstances, pathological changes can induce conditions that resemble the symptoms caused by the external pathogenic influences. In such cases, one speaks of "internal dampness," "internal cold," "internal heat," "internal wind," and so on.

Wind (Feng)

Wind is characterized by a sudden onset and quick subsidence, lesions that shift location, and aversion to drafts. When affecting the skin, wind diseases cause itching. Other wind disease symptoms may include involuntary movement (twitching, tremors, and convulsions) or the sensation of abnormal movement (vertigo and dizziness).

Cold (Han)

Cold diseases are characterized by sensations of chills and or cold, muscular contraction, and localized pain that worsens with exposure to cold.

Dampness (Shi)

Dampness is associated with lingering illness, heaviness of body and limbs, or headache that feels as if the head is tightly bound. There may be turbidity in body excretions, such as leucorrhea, turbid urine, and exudates from skin lesions. There can be sensations of fullness or distension in the abdomen, loss of appetite, nausea, vomiting, and loose stools, and in some cases, accumulation of fluids in the body, as in edema.

Dryness (Zao)

Dryness manifests as dry mouth, dry nose, dry throat, and dry cough.

Heat (Re)

Heat manifests as fever, thirst, scanty concentrated urine, constipation, a red tongue with yellow or no coating, and a rapid pulse. There may also be low fever in the afternoon, sensation of heat in the palms and soles, malar flush, and night sweating.

Fire (Huo)

Fire represents a stronger degree of heat and can manifest as acute inflammation and localized redness, swelling, sensation of heat, and pain, fever, restlessness, thirst, foul breath, bitterness in the mouth, ulceration of the tongue, and constipation, bleeding (epistaxis, hematuria, and so on), and a dark red tongue with a yellow, prickly coating, and rapid replete pulse. Diseases caused by endogenous fire are similar to those caused by endogenous heat, but may be accompanied by irritability and insomnia.

Endogenous Pathogens: The Seven Emotions (Qi Qing)

TCM treats excessive or unbalanced emotions as disease-causing factors because, through the systemic correspondences of five-phase theory, they are directly related to the zangfu organ systems. Each of the five zang is keyed to one emotion. The emotions are held to directly affect the movement of qi in specific ways which, like the six evils, may become pathogenic under given circumstances. Emotions are a natural part of human existence, and no human being is above experiencing them. Under normal circumstances, emotions occur in response to outside stimuli, produce an effect, and pass quickly. Emotions become the cause of disease only when they are intense, violent, or continue for long periods. This is sometimes termed "over-excitement of the emotions" in that the emotions exceed the adaptive, regulatory capability of the body. They can impair zangfu function, perturb the qi dynamic, and upset the yinyang balance, thus leading to the development of pathological conditions.

Because they are generated from within, emotions readily injure the zangfu. Each of the emotions is keyed to one of the zang, which it said to injure directly when in excess: euphoria injures the heart, anger injures the liver, sadness injures the lung, worry injures the spleen, and fear and fright injure the kidney. In addition, those organ systems directly in charge of mental/emotional activity, i.e., the heart and the liver, are affected by all pathological affects. The liver is directly in charge of coursing and discharging the emotions; a deterioration of this function causes the emotions to become more extreme. On the other hand, because the heart is the seat of mental activities, impairment or obstruction of this function will cause mania and depression.

The emotions perturb the movement of qi. Each of the emotions causes qi to move in a particular way, disturbing the qi dynamic on which the body depends to maintain harmony and balance. The disturbances of qi flow brought on by the emotions are summarized in table and explained later.

1. Anger induces qi to flow upward: The liver is the zang most readily affected by anger. When this happens, liver qi flows upward in excess, causing blood to move pathologically in this direction as well. This will manifest as a red face and eyes, dizziness and vertigo, distending pain of the head, or even sudden coma or syncope. Sometimes, hematemesis and diarrhea may also be observed as a result of blood following the adverse upward qi flow or a counterflow that attacks the spleen.

2. Euphoria relaxes the flow of qi: Euphoria is excessive joy. Under normal circum stances, joy is desirable in that it promotes the harmonious flow of qi and blood. However, taken to excess, it causes poor concentration and mania.

3. Sadness consumes qi: Affecting the lung and its command of breathing, sadness as a pathogenic factor manifests as chest oppression and a demoralized attitude. Crying and weeping exhaust the qi and cause lassitude.

4. Worry causes qi to accumulate: Discursive thought requires qi to become fixed. When it becomes lengthy or intense, thinking easily becomes worry and causes qi to stagnate. Worry most readily injures the spleen, and thus, the manifestations of injury by worry include poor appetite, abdominal distension, constipation, and diarrhea.

Table: Effect of the emotions on the movement of qi.

Emotion	Effect
Anger	Qi ascends
Euphoria	Qi relaxes
Worry	Qi accumulates
Sadness	Qi consumes
Fear	Qi descends
Fright	Qi disperses and moves recklessly

5. Fear causes *qi* to flow downward: Because the kidney is the *zang* in charge of urination and defecation, when fear injures it, there will be incontinence. Other manifestations include pain and weakness in the legs and knees as the function of the kidney to nourish the bones is impaired.

6. Fright causes *qi* to disperse: Sudden fear has the effect of causing the *qi* to col- lapse. This is seen as palpitations, anxiety or distress, and an inability to concentrate. Because emotional overexcitation causes a breakdown of the normal flow of qi, it will invariably cause stagnation. Over time, any obstruction or accumulation of qi leads to internal heat and fire. This is commonly seen in the clinic. Patients with long-term emotional problems usually display some of the symptoms associated with the fire pathogen. Key diagnostic signs are a red or crimson, dry tongue, possibly with a swollen and red tip, and a rapid and slippery pulse.

By the same token, emotions may also worsen a preexisting disease through their alter- ation of the qi dynamic. For example, a patient with hypertension (a disease caused by excessive rising of liver yang due to deficiency of both kidney and liver yin) may suffer from sudden coma or syncope, or even paralysis, after an incident of sudden and vio- lent rage. This is because the liver is readily affected by anger, and sudden anger will induce rising of liver yang.

Conversely, as body, mind, and emotions are an integral and indivisible unit, it is equal- ly likely for the process to occur in reverse, i.e., instead of the emotions causing disease, an organic disturbance may cause alteration of the emotions. For example, a state of protracted fear and anxiety will damage and weaken the kidney. On the other hand, if there is a deficiency of the kidney, due to having had multiple pregnancies and child- births, the condition may also manifest with abnormal states of fear and anxiety. Fre- quently, a vicious cycle is established, where the emotion will feed the organic imbal- ance, which, in turn, favors the imbalanced emotional state that worsens or aggravates it, such as when a liver imbalance makes a person irritable, which in turn aggravates the liver imbalance.

When thinking of the emotions as pathogenic influences, they are said to damage the interior and perturb the flow of qi of the zangfu. They arise and are keyed to the zang- fu and, under normal circumstances, will cause no damage as they are depurated by the liver's coursing and discharging. However, in excess, each of the emotions can af- fect one or more of the zangfu, causing pathological changes. Conversely, pathological changes in one of the zangfu may make one more prone to the emotion keyed to the affected organ system, which can create a vicious cycle of reinforcing disease-causing conditions.

Therapeutic Principles

Therapeutic principles are the criteria of treating all diseases. Formulated under the guidance of the concept of holism and treatment based on syndrome differentiation, they are significant for clinically guiding the determination of therapeutic methods, prescription and drugs.

Therapeutic principles are different from therapies. Guided by the former, the latter refers to the therapeutic rules and methods in accordance with various syndromes. Therapeutic rules are the criteria of classified treatment, and give specific guidance to therapeutic methods. They include diaphoresis, emesis, purgation, mediating, warming, heat-clearing, resoluting and reinforcing, also known as "major therapeutic rules". Extensively used in clinical practice, these eight rules are on the highest level among therapeutic rules. Whereas, therapeutic methods are those specific for various syndromes, limited in the range of therapeutic rules, such as nourishing blood to induce tranquilization, and releasing superficies with pungent-warm drugs, etc. Under the guidance of therapies, therapeutic measures should be further selected and determined, including oral use of drugs, acupuncture, tuina, external application, fumigation and washing.

Search for the Fundamental Cause of Disease in Treatment

It means to find the fundamental cause of a disease and focus the treatment on it. Reflecting the concept of holism and treatment based on syndrome differentiation, it is also a universal principle in traditional Chinese medicine when applying treatment to disease.

It includes routine treatment, contrary treatment and treating the fundamental and incidental aspects.

Routine Treatment and Contrary Treatment

Routine Treatment

It refers to the treatment of disease adverse to its manifestations (symptoms and signs), also known as "adverse treatment", applicable to disease with nature in conformity with its manifestations. For example, warm syndrome is marked by warm manifestations, cold syndrome by cold manifestations, deficiency syndrome by deficiency manifestations, and excess syndrome by excess manifestations. Since the nature (cold, hot, tonifying, purgative, etc.) and the action tendency of drugs are opposite to the manifestations of disease, it is accordingly known as "adverse treatment". Additionally, in clinic practice, manifestations of most disease are in conformity with the nature of disease, so treatment adverse to manifestations of disease is a general therapeutic principle, termed as "routine treatment".

Treat Cold with Heat

It means that the cold syndrome, with cold manifestations, should be treated with warming or hot formula. For example, releasing superficies with pungent-warm drugs is used to treat wind-cold syndrome of exterior type, and warming interior with pungent-hot drugs to treat the interior cold syndrome.

Treat Heat with Cold

It means that the heat syndrome, with heat manifestations, should be treated with cold or cool formula. For example, releasing superficies with pungent-cool drugs is used to treat wind-heat syndrome of exterior type, and relieving interior with bitter-cold drugs to treat heat accumulation in the stomach and intestines.

Treat Deficiency by Tonifying

It means that deficiency of healthy qi, with deficiency manifestations, should be treated with tonifying and replenishing formula. For example, replenishing qi is used to treat the qi deficiency syndrome, and nourishing yin to treat the yin deficiency syndrome.

Treat Excess by Purging

It means that excess of pathogenic qi, with excess manifestations, should be treated with offensive purgative formula. For example, dispelling retained water is used to treat internal retention of water, and promoting digestion and removing food stagnation to treat food stagnation.

Contrary Treatment

It refers to the treatment of disease agreeable to its manifestations, also known as "agreeable treatment", applicable to complicated morbid states in which the nature of disease is not completely in conformity with its manifestations, or even marked by false manifestations. For example, heat syndrome is marked by cold manifestations, cold syndrome by heat manifestations, deficiency syndrome by excess manifestations, and excess syndrome by deficiency manifestations. Since the nature (cold, hot, tonifying, purgative, etc.) and the action tendency of formula are agreeable to the manifestations of disease, it is accordingly known as "agreeable treatment". Since this kind of case is seldom seen in clinic practice and opposite to routine treatment, it is termed as "contrary treatment".

Treat Heat with Heat

It means that diseases with manifestations of false heat should be treated with warm or hot formula or measures, applicable to the syndrome of true cold with false heat caused by exuberant yin with repelled yang. For example, in Shanghan Lun (Treaties on Cold-Induced Disease), warm and hot formula, namely Tong Mai Si Ni Tang (Tongmaisini Decoction), is used to treat this case. When the pathogenic qi of yin cold is cleared away, false heat will disappear subsequently.

Treat Cold with Cold

It means that diseases with manifestations of false cold should be treated with cold or cool formula or measures, applicable to the syndrome of true heat with false cold caused by exuberant yang with repelled yin. For example, in Shanghan Lun (Treaties on Cold-Induced Disease), cold and cool formula, namely Baihu Tang (Baihu decoction), is used to treat heat syncope caused by exuberant internal yang with yin repelled externally. When the pathogenic qi of yang heat is cleared away, false cold will disappear subsequently.

Treat Stuffiness with Tonic

It means that diseases with manifestations of stuffiness should be treated with tonifying and replenishing formula or measures, also known as "relieving stuffiness with tonic", applicable to the syndrome of stuffiness and stagnation caused by deficiency. For example, abdominal distension and fullness, caused by deficiency of spleen and stomach and qi stagnation, is treated by invigorating spleen and replenishing qi. When the spleen and stomach function normally in transportation, distension and fullness will disappear spontaneously. For more examples, constipation due to qi deficiency, dysuria due to kidney deficiency and amenorrhea due to blood exhaustion can all be treated by "relieving stuffiness with tonic" with tonifying and replenishing formula.

Treat Diarrhea with Purgative

Classification	Concept	Contents	Indication	Common character	
Routine treatment	The routine treatment of disease adverse to its manifestations also known as adverse treatment.	Treat cold with heat.	Cold syndrome.	Nature of disease is in conformity with is manifestation.	Treatment focuses on the nature of disease.
		Treat heat with cold.	Heat syndrome.		
		Treat deficiency by tonifying.	Deficiency syndrome.		
		Treat excess by purging.	Excess syndrome.		
Contrary treatment	The treatment of disease agreeable to its manifestation, also known as agreeable treatment.	Treat hat with heat.	Symptom of true cold with false deat.	Nature of disease is not completely in conformity with its manifestations.	
		Treat cold with cold.	Symptom of true heat with flase cold.		
		Treat stuffiness with tonic.	Symptom of true deficiency with false excess.		
		Treat diarrhea with purgatives.	Symptom of true excess with false deficiency.		

It means that diseases with manifestations of diarrhea should be treated with purgative formula or measures, applicable to the syndrome of diarrhea caused by stagnation of excess pathogens. For example, dysentery caused by stagnation of damp-heat in the large intestine abdominal distension and fullness is treated by clearing heat and draining heat as well as promoting qi flow and relieving stagnation. When damp and heat are cleared away, diarrhea will be stopped spontaneously. For more examples, diarrhea caused by dyspepsia and metrorrhagia and metrostaxis caused by stagnant blood can be treated respectively with digestive formula and blood-activating and stasis-resoving formula, which are the so-called "treat diarrhea with purgative".

Routine treatment is different from contrary treatment. The former is the routing treatment of disease adverse to its manifestations, applicable to disease with nature in conformity with its manifestations. The latter is contrary to the routine treatment but agreeable to manifestations of disease, applicable to complicated morbid states in which the nature of disease is not completely in conformity with its manifestations or even marked by false manifestations. Besides, routine treatment and contrary treatment share some common points, i.e. both of them focus on the nature of disease, so they both pertain to search for the fundamental of disease in treatment.

Treating Fundamental Aspect and Incidental Aspect

The fundamental and the incidental are two relatively opposite concepts. Their relationship is often used to generalize and explain the essence and the outward appearance. In traditional Chinese medicine, it is mainly used to illuminate the relationship between the primary and the secondary of various contradictions during the course of a disease. Generally speaking, the fundamental is primary contradiction or the primary aspect of a contradiction; while the incidental is secondary contradiction or the secondary aspect of a contradiction. In the course of a disease, its fundamental aspect and incidental aspect are determined by the development of the disease. For example, healthy qi is the fundamental aspect, and pathogenic qi the incidental aspect; the cause of disease is the fundamental aspect, and the symptoms incidental aspect; primary disease is the fundamental aspect, and secondary disease the incidental aspect.

Application of Treating Fundamental Aspect and Incidental Aspect

Disease has aspects of the fundamental and the incidental, or aspects of the primary and the secondary, and treatment can be carried out in order of time and urgency. Only by resolving the primary contradiction of a disease first after distinguishing the fundamental from the incidental and the primary from the secondary, can the essence of treatment be grasped: Treating incidental aspect, treating fundamental aspect, or treating both fundamental and incidental aspects.

Treating Fundamental Aspect in Case of Lesser Urgency

For chronic disease or acute disease at the recovery stage, treatment should be focused on the fundamental aspect of a disease, for the incidental aspect usually originates from the fundamental aspect. When the fundamental aspect is cured, the incidental aspect will disappear subsequently. Take cough due to tuberculosis for example. Yin deficiency of the lung and kidney are the fundamental aspects, while cough is the incidental aspect. Therefore, it should he treated by nourishing yin of the lung and kidney, which is to treat the fundamental aspect. When yin fluid of the lung and kidney moistens, cough will be relieved naturally.

Treating Incidental Aspect in Case of Urgency

When the incidental aspect of a disease is so urgent and serious that it affects the treatment of the fundamental aspect and endangers patient's life, treatment should be focused on it first. For example, hematorrhea of any reason should be treated by arresting bleeding first, which is to treat the incidental aspect. When bleeding is stopped, its fundamental aspect should be further searched for and treated later on. It is thus evident that treating incidental aspect in case of urgency is actually an expedient measure. It means to create favorable conditions for the treatment of the fundamental aspect and aims to finally better treat its fundamental aspect.

Moreover, for those who suffer from old chronic disease and newly contract other pathogens, the old disease is the fundamental aspect and the new contraction is the incidental aspect. Although the incidental aspect is not very urgent, if not treated first, it will affect the treatment of the fundamental aspect. Therefore, the new contraction should be treated ahead of the old one.

Treating both Fundamental and Incidental Aspects

When the incidental and fundamental aspects of a disease are both serious or both not urgent, treatment should be concentrated on both fundamental and incidental aspects. Take common cold caused by qi deficiency for example. Qi deficiency is the fundamental aspect, and cold is the incidental aspect. Then simply replenishing qi will cause stagnation of pathogenic qi and cold cannot be cured; simply releasing superficies will impair healthy qi. Only by replenishing qi and releasing superficies, or by treating both fundamental and incidental aspects, can cold get relieved. Thus, the principle of treating both fundamental and incidental aspects can be applied to diseases complicated with coexistence of exterior and interior syndromes as well as mixture of deficiency and excess.

Reinforcing the Healthy and Eliminating the Pathogenic

Struggle between the healthy and pathogenic qi determines the development of a disease. With preponderance of pathogenic qi and decline of healthy qi, disease will progress; with preponderance of healthy qi and decline of pathogenic qi, disease will regress. To change the relative strength of pathogenic and healthy qi and to promote recovery of disease, the healthy qi should be reinforced and the pathogenic qi should be eliminated.

Concepts and Relationships

Reinforcing the Healthy

It refers to tonify the healthy qi, build up constitutions, and improve the body's resistance against disease and recovery ability. it is mainly applied to deficiency syndrome, which means to "treat deficiency by tonifying". Such therapeutic methods as replenishing qi, nourishing blood and yin, and warming yang are all guided by this principle. The specific measures of reinforcing the healthy are diverse, including drugs, acupuncture and moxibustion, qigong, regulation of emotions and diet, physical exercise, etc.

Eliminating the Pathogenic

It refers to remove the pathogenic qi and to relieve the invasion and impairment of pathogenic qi. It is mainly applied to excess syndrome, which means to "treat excess by purging". Such therapeutic methods as diaphoresis, emesis, purgation, resolving food stagnation, resolving phlegm, activating blood, dispersing cold, clearing away heat and dispelling dampness are all guided by this principle. The specific measures of eliminating the pathogenic are also diverse, including drugs, acupuncture and moxibustion, tuina, etc.

Relationship between Reinforcing the Healthy and Eliminating the Pathogenic

Reinforcing the healthy and eliminating the pathogenic are complementary. Reinforcing the healthy helps to tonify healthy qi and to prevent and dispel pathogenic qi, i.e. "when healthy qi is exuberant, pathogenic qi will be dispelled naturally"; whereas, eliminating the pathogenic helps to remove pathogenic factors and to conserve and recover healthy qi, i.e., "when pathogenic qi is driven out of the body, healthy qi will recover naturally". Thus, reinforcing the healthy helps to eliminate pathogenic qi, while eliminating the pathogenic helps to reinforce healthy qi. But they are two completely different therapeutic principles. Drugs of reinforcing the healthy tend to make pathogenic qi retain in the body, while drugs of eliminating the pathogenic tend to impair the healthy qi. So clinically, the increase or decrease of healthy or pathogenic qi should be first carefully analyzed to decide whether to reinforce the healthy, or to eliminate the pathogenic, or to combine both together.

Application of Reinforcing the Healthy and Eliminating the Pathogenic

Generally speaking, reinforcing the healthy is used for deficiency syndrome, while eliminating the pathogenic is used for excess syndrome. If a syndrome is mixed with deficiency of healthy qi and excess of pathogenic qi, it should he treated by both reinforcing the healthy and eliminating the pathogenic. During the treatment, attention should be paid to differentiate what is primary from what is secondary and what is urgent from what is less urgent, so that reinforcing the healthy and eliminating the pathogenic can be taken up in order of importance and priority.

Single Application

Reinforcing the Healthy

It is applicable to deficiency syndrome in which deficiency of healthy qi is the primary contradiction and meanwhile pathogenic qi is not exuberant. It is realized by tonifying and replenishing. For example, qi deficiency is treated by replenishing qi, blood deficiency by tonifying blood, yang deficiency by strengthening yang, yin deficiency by replenishing yin, etc.

Eliminating the Pathogenic

It is applicable to excess syndrome in which exuberance of pathogenic qi is the primary contradiction and meanwhile healthy qi does not decline. It is realized by purgation. For example, excess of exterior pathogens is treated by inducing sweating to release superficies, phlegm, saliva and retained food due to pathogens retained in the chest are treated by emesis, heat accumulation in the stomach and intestines is treated by purgation with bitter cold drugs, accumulation of heat and fire is treated by clearing away heat and purging fire, etc.

Combined Application

Reinforcing the Healthy Combined with Eliminating the Pathogenic

Reinforcing the healthy is the main focus of treatment and eliminating the pathogenic is also taken into consideration. It is applicable to syndromes with deficiency of healthy qi as the primary contradiction and exuberance of pathogenic qi as the secondary contradiction. For such syndromes, if healthy qi is not reinforced, pathogenic qi will become more savage; whereas, if pathogenic qi is not eliminated, healthy qi will be impaired further. Therefore, reinforcing the healthy combined with eliminating the pathogenic should be used. For exampte, heart vessel obstruction syndrome caused by deficiency of heart qi should he treated by tonifying and replenishing heart qi combined with activating blood and resolving stasis.

Eliminating the Pathogenic Combined with Reinforcing the Healthy

Eliminating the pathogenic is the main focus of treatment and reinforcing the healthy is also taken into consideration. It is applicable to syndromes with exuberance of pathogenic qi as the primary contradiction and deficiency of healthy qi as the secondary contradiction. For such syndromes, if pathogenic qi is not eliminated, healthy qi will be impaired further; whereas, if healthy qi is not reinforced, pathogenic qi will become more savage. Therefore, treatment should be focused on reinforcing the healthy and simultaneously be combined with eliminating the pathogenic. For example, damage of yin by heat should be treated by clearing away heat combined with nourishing yin.

Alternate Application

Reinforcing the Healthy Prior to Eliminating the Pathogenic

It is applicable to syndromes of deficiency of healthy qi with excess of pathogenic qi, in which healthy qi cannot withstand attack. Though there is excess of pathogenic qi, healthy qi should be first reinforced by tonifying, as it is too weak to withstand attack. After healthy qi becomes strong enough to withstand attack, the pathogenic can be eliminated then. Take patients with the syndrome of helminthic accumulation for example. Since the spleen qi has already declined to extremes so that it cannot withstand parasiticides, healthy qi should be first reinforced by invigorating spleen and replenishing qi. When deficiency of the spleen is gradually relieved, measures should be taken to dispel helminthic accumulation then.

Eliminating the Pathogenic Prior to Reinforcing the Healthy

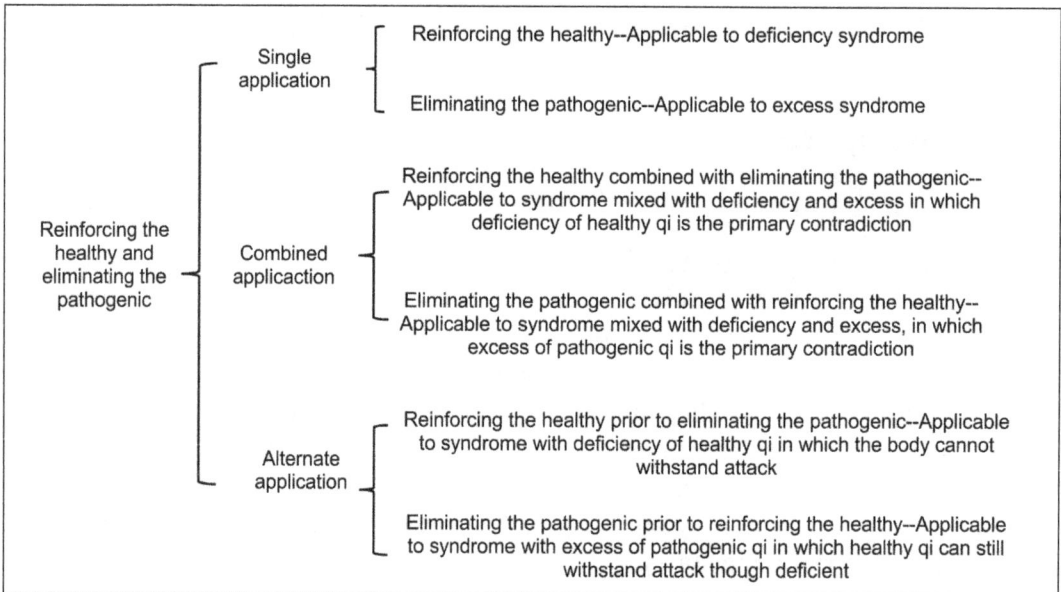

It is applicable to syndromes of excess of pathogenic qi with deficiency of healthy qi and, in which pathogenic qi needs eliminating urgently and healthy qi can still withstand attack. Though healthy qi is deficient, it can still withstand attack. So pathogenic qi should be first eliminated by purgation, and then regulating and tonifying can be taken up. Take blood deficiency caused by stagnant blood, metrorrhagia and metrostaxis for example. If stagnant blood is not removed, metrorrhagia and metrostaxis cannot be stopped and blood deficiency will worse. So, stagnant blood should be dispelled by activating blood and dispelling stasis and then measures should be taken to tonify and nourish blood.

Regulating Yin and Yang

The fundamental mechanism of disease is disharmony of yin and yang. Therefore, regulating yin and yang for the purpose of reestablishing coordination and balance is a cardinal therapeutic principle.

Reducing Excess

It means to treat syndromes with preponderance of yin or yang by reducing excessive yin pathogens or yang pathogens. Preponderance of yang causes the syndrome of excess heat, and should be treated by "treating heat with cold", i.e. cold-cool drugs are used to clear away and purge yang heat, preponderance of yin causes the syndrome of excess cold, and should be treated by "treating cold with heat", i.e. warm-hot drugs are used to dispel yin cold.

Supplementing Insufficiency

It means to treat syndromes with decline of yin or yang by supplementing insufficient yin or yang. Decline of yin or yang includes deficiency of yin, deficiency of yang and deficiency of both yin and yang. Therefore, treatment should be determined flexibly according to individual conditions.

Nourishing Yin

It is applicable to yin deficiency. Since deficient, yin cannot restrict yang and yang becomes preponderant. As a result, a syndrome of deficiency-heat occurs, which should be treated by nourishing yin so as to restrict yang, i.e. "strengthening the governor of water to restrict hyperactivity of yang".

Tonifying Yang

It is applicable to yang deficiency. Since deficient, yang cannot restrict yin and yin becomes preponderant. As a result, a syndrome of deficiency-cold occurs, which should be treated by tonifying yang so as to restrict yin. i.e. "supplementing the source of fire to eliminate preponderance of yin".

Supplementing both Yin and Yang

It exactly means to both nourish yin and tonify yang, and is applicable to deficiency of both yin and yang. Yin deficiency should be treated by nourished yin, yang deficiency by tonifying yang, and deficiency of both yin and yang by supplementing both yin and yang. When this principle is applied to treatment, attention should be paid to differentiate what is primary from what is secondary and what is early from what is late, so that nourishing yin and tonifying yang can be taken up in order of importance.

Yang impairment involving yin is marked by deficiency of both yin and yang, with yang deficiency as the primary contradiction of disease. It should be treated by "treating yin for yang", namely tonifying yang supplemented by nourishing yin. Yin impairment involving yang is marked by deficiency of both yin and yang, with yin deficiency as the primary contradiction of disease. It should be treated by "treating yang for yin", namely nourishing yin supplemented by tonifying yang.

Moreover, due to the relativity of the implication of yin and yang, all pathological changes can be generalized by disharmony of yin and yang. Therefore, in a broad sense, the following therapeutic methods belong to the scope of regulating yin and yang, releasing superficies and relieving interior, emesis and purgation, raising the lucid and dropping the turbid, warming cold and clearing heat, reinforcing deficiency and reducing excess, regulating visceral functions, regulating qi and blood, etc.

Regulating Qi and Blood

Qi and blood are the essential substances for the maintenance of life activities and also the material basis of functional activities of various tissues and organs such as viscera and meridians. Disorders of qi and blood will involve the whole body, while pathological changes of any part of the body will cause disorders of qi and blood. Therefore, it is an important therapeutic principle.

Regulating Qi

Tonifying Qi

It is applicable to qi deficiency. Qi of the human body comes from innate qi, food nutrients and clear qi of nature, and is formed by qi transformation of the lungs, spleen, stomach and kidney. Innate defects, required malnutrition and the functional disorders of the lung, kidneys, spleen and stomach can all lead to qi deficiency. Therefore, tonifying qi is to tonify and replenish the kidney, spleen, stomach and lung. Since the spleen and stomach play a major role in the generation of required qi, tonifying qi attaches great importance to qi of the spleen and stomach.

Regulating Qi Movement

It refers to regulate the movements of qi, including ascending, descending, exiting and entering, applicable to syndromes caused by disorders of qi movement. For example, qi stagnation should be treated by promoting flow of qi, reversed flow of qi by driving qi downward, sinking of qi by raising qi, etc.

Harmonizing Blood

Tonifying Blood

It is applicable to syndromes of blood deficiency. Since blood originates from food nutrients and is generated by qi transformation of the spleen, stomach, heart, kidney, liver, etc. So tonifying blood is mainly to regulate and tonify functions of these viscera. And as the generative source of qi and blood, the spleen and stomach play a critical role in the generation of qi and blood. Consequently, tonifying blood attaches great importance to regulate and nourish the spleen and stomach.

Cooling Blood

It is applicable to syndromes of blood heat. Blood heat can be caused by deficiency and excess as well as external contraction and internal injuries, clinically marked by fever, hemorrhage, upset, etc. Therefore, cooling blood should be flexibly used in clinical treatment. For example, high fever caused by blood heat should be treated by cooling blood and clearing heat; hemorrhage caused by blood heat should be treated by cooling blood to stop bleeding; disturbance of heart by blood heat should be treated by cooling blood to tranquilize mind.

Activating Blood

It is applicable to syndromes of stagnant blood. Stagnant blood can be caused by various reasons, including blood cold, blood heat, qi deficiency, reversed flow of qi, yin deficiency, hemorrhage, excessive emotional stimulation, traumatic injuries, etc. Therefore, activating blood should be flexibly used in clinical treatment. For example, stagnant blood caused by blood cold should be treated by warming meridians and dispersing cold to promote blood circulation; stagnant blood caused by qi deficiency should be treated by tonifying qi and activating blood.

Regulating the Relationship between Qi and Blood

Qi and blood are closely related to and complement each other. So pathologically, they usually affect each other. For example, qi disorders involve blood, blood disorders involve qi, etc. Therefore, the relationship between qi and blood should be regulated.

Regulating Qi Supplemented by Regulating Blood

Since qi generates blood, deficiency of both qi and blood, caused by insufficient generation of blood due to qi deficiency, should be treated by tonifying qi supplemented by tonifying blood. Since qi promotes the circulation of blood, blood stagnation caused by qi stagnation should be treated by promoting the flow of qi supplemented by activating blood and resolving stasis; stagnant blood, caused by failure of deficient qi, should be treated by tonifying qi supplemented by activating blood. Since qi governs blood, so hemorrhage caused by qi deficiency should be treated by tonifying qi supplemented by stopping bleeding with astringents.

Regulating Blood Supplemented by Regulating Qi

Since blood nourishes qi, qi deficiency resulted from blood deficiency should he treated by nourishing blood supplemented by tonifying qi; Since blood transports qi, deficiency of both qi and blood resulted from chronic hemorrhage should be treated by stopping bleeding and nourishing blood supplemented by tonifying qi. However, qi prostration after blood prostration resulted from hemorrhage should be treated first by replenishing qi and stopping bleeding, and then by tonifying blood and replenishing qi when the disease is somewhat relieved.

Treatment in Seasonal Conditions, Local Conditions and Patient's Individuality

It means that therapeutic principles should be determined according to seasonal, local and individual conditions, also known as "treatment in accordance with three factors". Traditional Chinese medicine holds that the occurrence, development and change of disease are influenced by various internal and external factors. Therefore, in clinical practice, seasonal climates, geographic environment and individual differences should be all taken into account, and individual differences should be all taken into account, and appropriate methods should be chosen according to specific conditions.

Treatment in Accordance with Seasonal Conditions

It refers to that therapeutic principles should be determined according to features of seasonal climates.

Since seasonal variations of weather, from coolness and cold to warmness and heat, to a certain degree, influence physiology and pathology of the body, treatment and prescription should be different in different seasons. Different seasons, characterized by diverse features of climates, have different requirements for dosage as well as cold or hot nature of drugs. For example, in spring and summer when the weather changes from warm to hot and yang qi ascends, the interstices of the body become looser. During this period, even for external contraction of wind-cold, pungent-warm dispersing drugs, such as Ma Huang (Herba Ephedrae) and Gui Zhi (Ramulus Cinnamomi), should be used cautiously so as not to impair qi and yin due to excessive dispersion; in autumn and winter when the weather turns cold from cool and yin becomes preponderant with decline of yang, the interstices become tighter and yang qi retreats interiorly. So drugs of cool or cold nature, such as Shi Gao (Gypsum Fibrosum) and Bo He (Herba Menthae), should be used cautiously to avoid impairment of yang qi.

Treatment in Accordance with Local Conditions

It refers to that therapeutic principles should be determined according to features of geographical environment.

Individuals in various geographic environments differ in constitutional features and pathological changes due to diverse climatic conditions and living habits. Accordingly, treatment and prescription should be suited to local conditions as well. For example, in the northwestern highlands of China, it is cold and dry, with scanty rainfall. So wind-cold and dryness are commonly seen and usually treated by pungent-moistening formula, while cold-cool-dry formula should be used with great care. In the southeastern coastal lowlands of China, it is hot and damp, with plentiful rainfall. So damp-heat is commonly seen and should be treated by heat clearing and damp-resolving drugs, while damp-inducing drugs of warm or hot nature should be used cautiously.

Treatment in Accordance with Patient's Individuality

It refers to that therapeutic principles should be determined according to features of patient's age, sex, constitutions, living habits and occupations.

Age

Individuals of different ages are characterized by different physiological functions and pathological changes. Due to deficient qi and blood as well as decline of physiological functions, the aged people often suffer from deficiency syndrome or syndrome of deficiency-excess in complexity, which should be mainly treated by tonifying methods. Even when there are excess pathogens, drastic drugs; large dosage and long-term treatment are not advisable. As to infants, they are vigorous in physiological functions, but their qi and blood are not sufficient enough and their viscera are tender and delicate. Consequently, they are likely to be affected by cold or heat as well as deficiency or excess syndromes. Therefore, the small dosage of drugs is advisable, and drastic tonifying o purgation is contraindicated.

Gender

Man and woman have different physiological features. Especially, women have menstruation, leukorrhea, pregnancy and delivery, which all need special attention. For example, during pregnancy, drugs of drastic purgation, breaking stagnant blood, slipperiness, migration and toxicity should be contraindicated or used with great care. After labour, deficiency of qi and blood, breast-feeding and lochia should be taken into account.

Constitutions

Different types of constitutions have direct effect on the occurrence of disease, and produce different responses to medicinal treatment. Therefore, in clinical treatment, constitutional factors should be taken into account. For example, for the same disease, individuals with constitutions of yin deficiency and yang excess should be treated with great care by drugs of warm, hot, pungent and dry nature; those with constitutions of yang deficiency and yin excess should contraindicate drugs of cold, cool and fresh nature; those of strong constitutions, benefited from strong tolerance, can be treated by drastic drugs with large dosage; those of weak constitutions, owed to poor tolerance, should be treated by mild drugs with small dosage.

In addition, in diagnosis and treatment, attention should be also paid to psychological states, occupational features, working conditions and living environment, for they are all related to the occurrence of disease.

Organs in Chinese Medicine

Modern quantum science as well as the ancient teachings of Chinese medicine say that everything is energy. Everything that makes up a human being, mind-body-spirit, correlates at an energetic level to something "external" in nature. We can use the vibrational frequency of nature and these principles of natural law to heal and balance our bodies and emotions.

This principle of interconnectedness also applies between different physical aspects of our bodies. For example, the Kidney organ correlates with the tissue of bone/teeth, the sensory taste of salt, the sensory organ of the ear, and the areas of the lower back, knees, and the heels/feet.

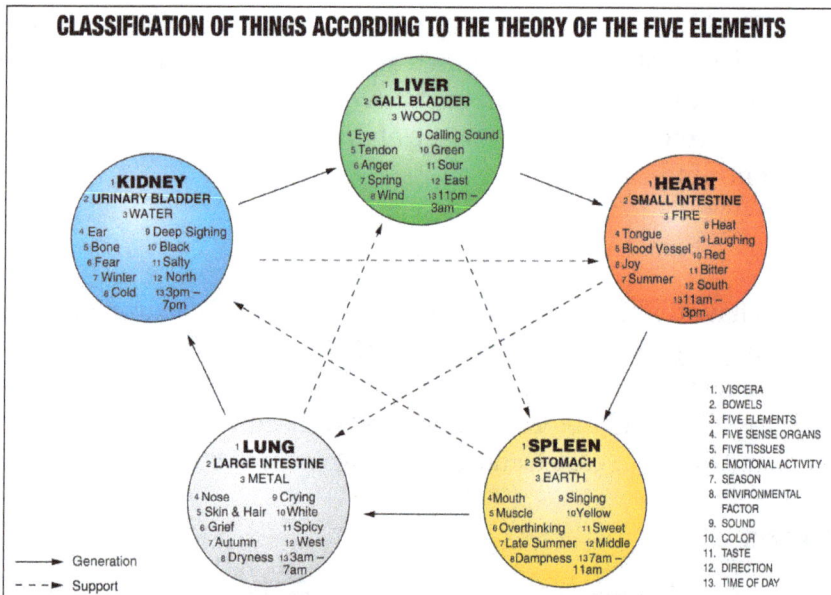

CLASSIFICATION OF THINGS ACCORDING TO THE THEORY OF THE FIVE ELEMENTS

Liver/Gallbladder according to Five Element Theory

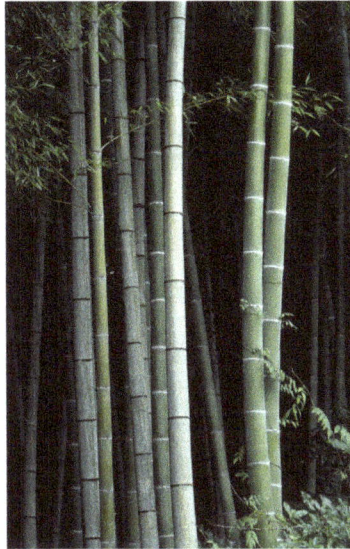

According to Traditional Chinese Medicine, the Liver is the organ responsible for the smooth flow of emotions as well as Qi and blood. It is the organ that is most affected by excess stress or emotions. The Liver's partner organ is the Gallbladder.

- The Liver is responsible for the smooth flow of Qi and blood in your body. It controls the volume and smooth flow of blood in your vessels and also stores the blood.

- The eyes are the sensory organ related to the Liver. If you have any eye issues, including blurry vision, red or dry eyes, itchy eyes, it may be a sign deep down that your Liver is not functioning smoothly.

- The tendons are the tissue associated with the Liver. TCM says that strength comes from the tendons, not muscles. Be like the cat that is strong, agile, and flexible, not the cow, which has huge muscles but little real strength.

- The taste that corresponds to and supports the Liver is sour. If you crave sour foods, that may be your Liver communicating that it needs an extra boost, so be sure to include high-quality vinegar and sweet and sour recipes in your diet.

- Anger is the emotion associated with the Liver. If you are often irritable, get angry easily, have trouble unwinding from the day's activities, have trouble reasoning or going with the flow and letting things go, you are experiencing a Liver function problem. Experiencing these emotions chronically or excessively can seriously unbalance the function of your Liver.

You can use these basic guidelines to begin to understand what organs may be asking for support. In the case of the Liver, if you constantly crave sour foods, or are under a great deal of stress and feel angered easily, then your Liver function needs support. Use these 'signs' to re-balance yourself.

Simple Tips for Everyday Liver Health

- Stay calm, especially during the spring. Don't get caught up in spring's intense new energies. Take things easy and go slow; take a nice long walk in the park or do other gentle exercises to relax your mind, body, and spirit. Let go of any stressful situations that you can, and if that's not possible, use some of the stress-relieving tips.

- Using a hairbrush with rounded bristles, hit your legs up and down the insides of your thighs and calves, starting at the ankles, for about five minutes. This gently stimulates your Liver meridian, allowing your qi to flow more freely and relaxing your Liver.

- Avoid alcohol. Because the Liver is responsible for metabolizing alcohol, drinking in moderation can go a long way towards preserving your Liver's energy and giving it a break.

- Engage in gentle exercise, such as swimming or walking, instead of hard and fast exercises which overwork or overstretch the tendons, causing them to eventually lose their flexibility, impacting the Liver function of being "flexible."

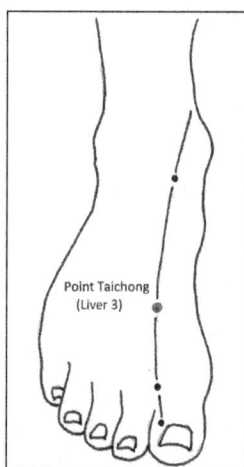

Point Taichong (Liver 3)

Acupressure for Liver Health

Rub the acupressure point called "Taichong" (Liver 3) which stimulates a key point on the Liver channel. It may be sore, but this means you're hitting all the right spots. You are unblocking your Liver Qi.

Try to rub this area every day. It's located on top of your foot where the big toe bone meets the second toe bone (about an inch back from the skin between these toes). Using your thumb, press and massage this spot on both feet (the meridians are on both sides of your body). You can also rub with your thumb moving forward along the inside of the big toe.

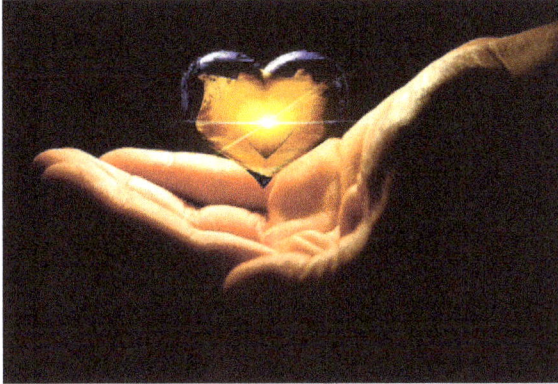

Heart/Small Intestine Health

The Heart, according to Chinese medicine, is the king of all organs. This means that all the other organs will sacrifice for the Heart. In other words, they will always give their energy to help the Heart maintain its balance. The Hearts partner is the Small Intestine.

The Stomach is the "child" of the Heart. If the Stomach is functioning well then the mother, the Heart is happy or less impacted. In this simple analogy we understand that Stomach energy must be in balance for Heart energy to be balanced.

The Five Element chart also shows us that the Liver is the "mother" of the Heart. When a person is under continual stress, Liver energy becomes compromised because one of its energetic functions is to smooth and regulate emotions. So when chronic stress or excessive emotion is experienced, the Liver cannot offer proper support to the Heart.

Because of these important relationships as described by Five Element Theory, if you want to really take care of your cardiovascular health, it's crucial to take care of your digestive organs, the Liver and the Stomach.

Read your Body from the Five Element Perspective

- Perspiration is the "fluid" of the Heart: Perspiration comes from body fluid, and the Heart controls bodily fluids. If you find you are perspiring excessively, it can signal a Qi or energy deficiency of the Heart. On the other hand, if you engage in activities that make you to sweat too much, this can cause a Qi deficiency of the Heart.

- The tongue is the sense organ related to the Heart: The condition of the Heart can be seen by observing the tongue. The tongue will be a healthy red color when this organ is in balance. If there is insufficient blood in the Heart, the tongue may appear pale. If there is blood stagnation, the tongue will reflect this with a dark purple color. Cracks or lines down the center of the tongue also indicate a potential Heart function issue.

- The blood vessels are considered the "tissue" of the Heart: Because the face has many blood vessels, the complexion reveals the state of the Heart. Like the tongue, a pale complexion can indicate insufficient blood, and an overly red face can signal excessive heat.

- Bitter is the taste associated with the Heart: If you find yourself craving bitter foods your Heart may be asking for support. Foods beneficial for the Heart are watermelon, plum tomatoes, broccoli and broccoli rabe.

Use these basic guidelines to listen to the body. In the case of the Heart, if you constantly crave bitter foods, or have difficulty sleeping it may be a sign that your Heart function needs support. Use these "signs" to re-balance yourself.

Simple Tips for Everyday Hearth Health

- Smile: Look in the mirror and smile at yourself. Do this multiple times until you feel a true smile emerging. Can you feel the difference between a pretend smile and and heartfelt one? Feel gratitude for yourself. Smiling stimulates the Heart and brings a sense of internal peace.

- Place your hands, one on top of the other over your chest area. Make a connection with your heart. Feel it beating. Make small circular motions.

- Before going to bed, allow your mind to wander. Begin to let all the business of the day drop out of your mind. Replace it instead with an image that is peaceful to you. With the palms of your hands placed gently over your heart, and a slight smile on your face, use this image to help you drift into a peaceful sleep.

- Go for a slow but steady walk. Place both hands behind you as you walk so your hands meet at your lower back.

Emergency First Aid for the Heart

If you experience any difficulty that may be associated with the heart, while waiting for help to arrive, try this simple tip, which provides stimulation to support your heart function. Open and close both hands, making sure your fingers curl down to touch the palms of your hands. Your middle fingers are the most important fingers to make a connection with the palms. Continue to open and close your hand for at least five minutes or as long as possible.

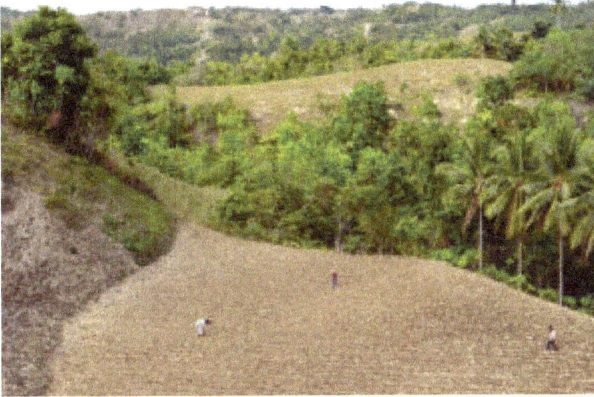

Stomach/Spleen Health

According to Traditional Chinese Medicine, the Stomach (and its partner the Spleen) is most affected by chronic worry, anxiety, or overthinking. Remember, the Stomach is responsible not only for digesting food and drink, but also for digesting your emotions and thoughts, keeping what nurtures your spirit and letting go of what doesn't.

The Stomach's element is Earth. Just as Mother Earth's job is to nurture growth and all living creatures, Stomach Qi is what "feeds" all the organs enough power to perform their jobs.

- The mouth is the sensory organ related to the Stomach. If you have any mouth issues, such as bleeding gums or bad breath, it may be a sign that your Stomach function is compromised.

- The muscles are the tissue associated with the Stomach. If your muscles are weak and underdeveloped, or if they cramp or tire easily, you may have a Stomach or Spleen dysfunction.

- The taste that corresponds to and supports the Stomach is sweet, according to Five Element theory. If you crave sweets, perhaps your Stomach needs support. The taste of sweet naturally supports the healthy function of your Stomach. Like a baby, the Stomach loves warm and hates cold. Reducing intake of cold drinks will support healthy Stomach function.

- Worry, anxiety, and overthinking are the emotions associated with the Stomach. If you constantly worry or over-think things (especially negative thoughts), get anxious easily, you may have a Stomach imbalance or function disorder. Experiencing any emotions chronically or excessively can damage Stomach and digestive health, as the digestive system processes not just the food you eat, but the thoughts and emotions that you internalize.

Foods to Support Stomach Health

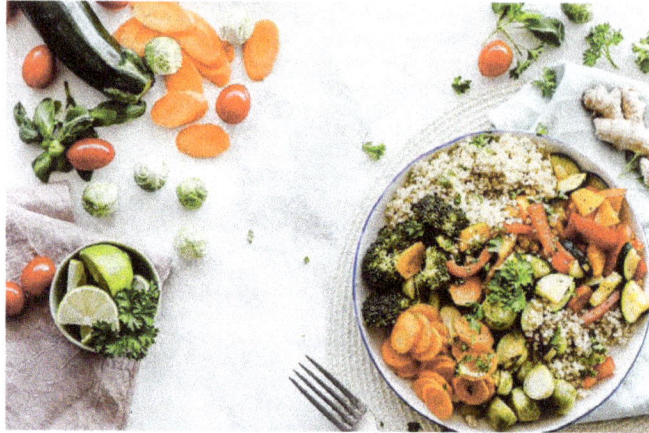

Many foods have an essence that supports the Stomach, especially yellow or orange foods, foods harvested in the late summer or root vegetables that grow directly in the ground. A TCM practitioner might regularly prescribe these foods for patients when trying to build strong Stomach function.

Simple Tips for Everyday Stomach Health

Some ways to take care of your Stomach:

- Don't worry, be happy: Worry, anxiety, and overthinking are the emotions that are associated with the Stomach and Spleen, and these emotions in excess have an especial impact on your digestive health.

- Eat mostly cooked or warm foods and beverages: Your Stomach is warmth loving by nature, so eating cold or raw foods (especially nuts and vegetables) and cold drinks can damage Stomach functioning over time. Raw fruit is okay as the essence of fruit is very light.

- Have your dinner by 6 or 7 pm at the latest: This gives your Stomach a chance to rest along with all your other organs! If you eat a lot or heavy foods at night, then you are making your Stomach work overtime when it should be resting.

Acupressure for Stomach Health

The zhongwan is the entire area from under your breastbone to above your navel. Massaging this area can help strengthen your digestive system and relieve symptoms such as nausea and lack of appetite.

Massage this area gently by placing one hand on top of the other and slowly making five circles. five more circles. Reverse direction and make five more circles. Repeat this routine for about five minutes.

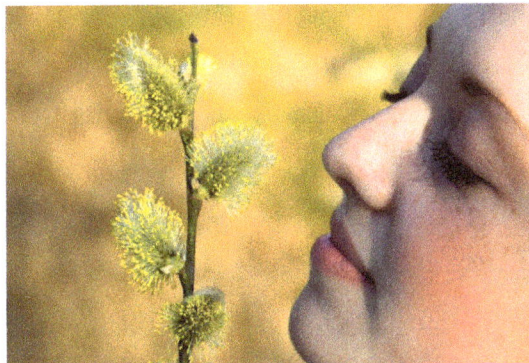

Lung/Large Intestine Health

What is the importance of the Lung to one's health? The Lung's major functions include maintaining healthy immune defenses against pathogens, as well as circulating Qi and fluids throughout the body.

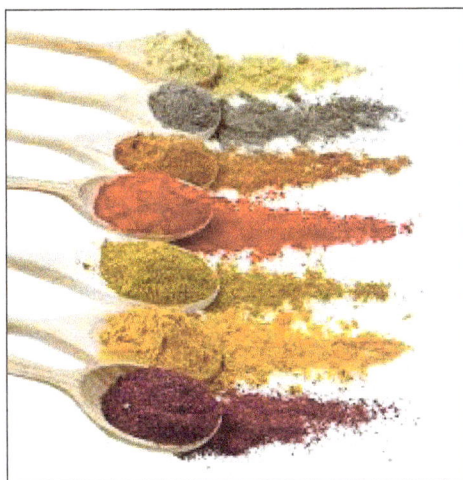

Emotionally and physically, the Lung (along with its organ partner, the Large Intestine), is responsible for helping you "let go" of whatever you don't need, from life experiences to emotions to actual metabolic by-products.

- Autumn is the season associated with the Lung and its partner, the Large Intestine. If you tend to catch colds or have allergies in the fall, it's important to take care of these organs.

- The nose is the sensory organ related to the Lung. Runny nose, sneezing, congested sinuses, loss of smell, are all symptoms of compromised Lung function.

- The skin is the tissue associated with the Lung. If you want to have healthy, clear, wrinkle-free skin, it's important to take care of the Lung and the Large Intestine.

- The taste that corresponds to and supports the Lung is spicy, according to Five Element theory.

- Sadness and grief are the emotions associated with the Lung and Large Intestine. If you cry easily or have trouble processing grief and loss, you may have an imbalance in your Lung energy.

Foods to Support Lung Health

Many foods have an essence that supports the Lung and its partner, the Large Intestine, especially spicy, white foods. An acupuncturist might regularly prescribe these foods for patients when trying to build strong Lung function.

Simple Tips for Everyday Lung Health

Some ways to take care of your Lung:

- Let go of things you no longer need and give yourself breathing room. Stimulate your Lung function by throwing out those twenty-year old clothes or notebooks from fifth grade.

- Bundle up in windy and cold weather, especially your chest and neck. Because part of the Lung's job is to protect you from pathogens, you can save Lung energy by covering up your skin.

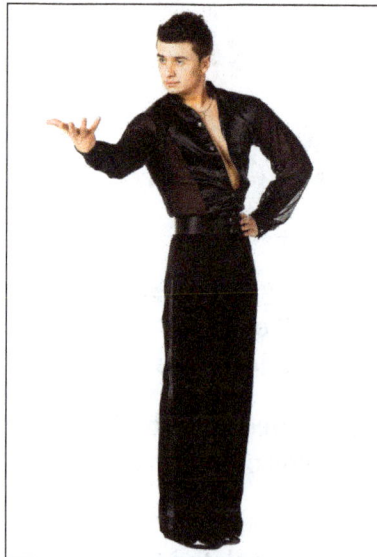

Qigong for Lung Health

Practice the most powerful Qigong movement from our popular wellness and weight loss program, "The Dragon Stands between Heaven and Earth".

Standing with feet shoulder-width apart and your knees slightly bent, raise your arms to chest level, and make two fists. Point your thumbs toward each other about six inches in front of you. Relax your arms and shoulders, but keep your hands at this height. Take a few deep breaths. Close your eyes, and imagine you are a dragon standing between Heaven and Earth.Hold this posture as long as you can. This not only strengthens Lung energy but also increases your overall energy levels in your body, giving you extra Qi for healing and living.

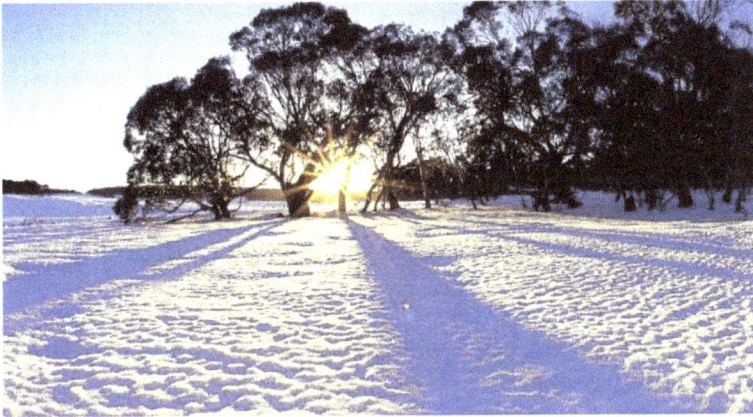

Kidney/Bladder Health

According to Traditional Chinese Medicine, the Kidney is the powerhouse of the body, supplying reserve energy to any organ running low on Qi. Its partner organ is the Bladder. The season associated with the Kidney is the Winter so it's especially important to slow down and conserve energy by getting more rest:

- The Kidney stores reserve energy called "pre-natal Qi" inherited from your parents. When another organ is low on energy, the Kidney sends it an extra Qi boost from this inheritance.

- The ears are the sensory organs related to the Kidney. Any ear problems, such as deafness, tinnitus, or ear infections are a signal from your body that the Kidney's energy needs extra support.

- The bone is the tissue associated with the Kidney. If the Kidney's energy is low, you may have symptoms such as osteoporosis, dental issues, or developmental issues.

- The taste that corresponds to and supports the Kidney is salt, according to the Five Element theory.

- Fear is the emotion associated with the Kidney. If you often have severe panic attacks, anxiety, and fear, your body may be trying to tell you that Kidney energy is running low or is imbalanced.

Foods to Support Kidney Health

Many foods have an essence that resonates with the Kidney. You may crave seafood, beans or bone soup. These are all foods that build strong Kidney function. Listen to the body, and eat what you are in the "mood" for.

Simple Tips for Everyday Kidney Health

Some ways to support your Kidney's energy:

- Stomp your feet, slowly and with flat feet, for about 5 minutes a day. This stimulates your Kidney's energy as the feet are associated with the Kidney and Bladder meridians, which run through the heel and to the sole of the foot.

- Rub your ears for several minutes a day. This simple massage strengthens Kidney function, as the ears are connected energetically to the Kidney organ and meridian.

- Stop energy drains. Conserve your energy by sleeping before midnight, resting when you're tired, and giving yourself permission to take a break and de-stress.

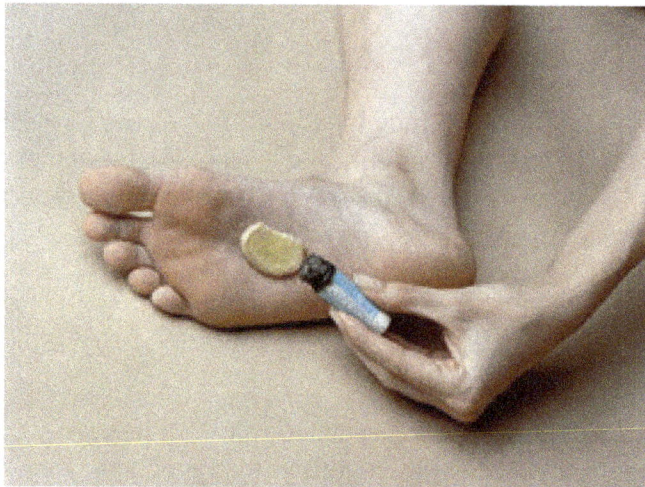

Acupressure for Kidney Health

Rub the acupressure point called "Yongquan" or "Gushing Spring" which stimulates a key point on the Kidney channel. It may be sore, but this means you're hitting the right spot to stimulate your body's energy foundation and relieve symptoms such as night sweats, hot flashes, tinnitus, hypertension, insomnia, anxiety, and headaches.

The yongquan is located at the exact center of the bottom of each foot. Starting with your left foot, massage this point as deeply as comfortable using your thumb or even a tennis ball—anything you have on hand.

Emotions in Traditional Chinese Medicine

In traditional Chinese medicine, emotions and physical health are intimately connected. Sadness, nervous tension and anger, worry, fear, and overwork are each associated with a particular organ in the body. For example, irritability and inappropriate anger can affect the liver and result in menstrual pain, headache, redness of the face and eyes, dizziness and dry mouth.

A diagnosis in traditional Chinese medicine is highly individualized. Once an organ system is identified, the unique symptoms of the patient determine the practitioner's treatment approach.

Using the liver again as an example, breast distension, menstrual pain, and irritability during menses are treated with certain herbs and acupuncture points. Headaches, dizziness, and inappropriate anger with redness of the face point to a different type of liver pattern and is treated in a different way.

What does the liver have to do with migraines? Organ systems in the traditional Asian sense may include the Western medical-physiological function, but are also part of a holistic body system. The liver, for example, ensures that energy and blood flow smoothly throughout the body. It also regulates bile secretion, stores blood, and is connected with the tendons, nails, and eyes.

By understanding these connections, we can see how an eye disorder such as conjunctivitis might be due to an imbalance in the liver, or excess menstrual flow may be due to dysfunction in the liver's blood-storing ability. Besides emotions, other factors such as dietary, environmental, lifestyle, and hereditary factors also contribute to the development of imbalances.

Spleen

- Emotions: Worry, dwelling or focusing too much on a particular topic, excessive mental work.

- Spleen Function: Food digestion and nutrient absorption. Helps in the formation of blood and energy. Keeps blood in the blood vessels. Connected with muscles, mouth, and lips. Involved in thinking, studying, and memory.

- Symptoms of Spleen Imbalance: Tired, loss of appetite, mucus discharge, poor digestion, abdominal distension, loose stools or diarrhea. Weak muscles, pale lips. Bruising, excess menstrual blood flow, and other bleeding disorders.

- Spleen Conditions: Spleen Qi Deficiency, Spleen Qi Descending, Spleen Yang Deficiency.

Lung

- Emotions: Grief, sadness, detached.

- Lung Function: Respiration forms energy from air, and helps to distribute it throughout the body. Works with the kidney to regulate water metabolism. Important in the immune system and resistance to viruses and bacteria. Regulates sweat glands and body hair, and provides moisture to the skin.

- Symptoms of Lung Imbalance: Shortness of breath and shallow breathing, sweating, fatigue, cough, frequent cold and flu, allergies, asthma, and other lung conditions.

- Lung Conditions: Lung Qi Deficiency, Lung Yin Deficiency, and Cold Damp Obstructing the Lungs.

Liver

- Emotions: Anger, resentment, frustration, irritability, bitterness, "flying off the handle".

- Liver Function: Involved in the smooth flow of energy and blood throughout the body. Regulates bile secretion, stores blood, and is connected with the tendons, nails, and eyes.

- Symptoms of Liver Imbalance: Breast distension, menstrual pain, headache, irritability, inappropriate anger, dizziness, dry, red eyes and other eye conditions, tendonitis.

- Liver Conditions: Liver Qi Stagnation, Liver Fire.

Heart

- Emotions: Lack of enthusiasm and vitality, mental restlessness, depression, insomnia, despair.

- Heart Function: Regulates the heart and blood vessels. Responsible for even and regular pulse. Influences vitality and spirit. Connected with the tongue, complexion, and arteries.

- Symptoms of Heart Imbalance: Insomnia, heart palpitations and irregular heartbeat, excessive dreaming, poor long-term memory, psychological disorders.

- Heart Conditions: Heart Yin and Heart Fire.

Kidney

- Emotions: Fearful, weak willpower, insecure, aloof, isolated.

- Kidney Function: Key organ for sustaining life. Responsible for reproduction, growth and development, and maturation. Involved with lungs in water metabolism and respiration. Connected with bones, teeth, ears, and head hair.

- Symptoms of Kidney Imbalance: Frequent urination, urinary incontinence, night sweats, dry mouth, poor short-term memory, low back pain, ringing in the ears, hearing loss, and other ear conditions. Premature gray hair, hair loss, and osteoporosis.

- Kidney Conditions: Kidney Yin Deficiency and Kidney Yang Deficiency.

Other TCM Conditions

- Blood Stagnation

- Blood Deficiency

- Stomach Heat

Using TCM

Since symptoms of these TCM syndromes in alternative medicine may be linked to a number of medical conditions, it's important to consult your physician if you have any health concerns. Self-treating a health condition and avoiding or delaying standard care may have serious consequences.

Six Climatic Factors

The six climatic factors are pathogenic wind, pathogenic cold, pathogenic summer-heat, pathogenic dampness, pathogenic dryness and pathogenic heat (fire).

Wind, cold, summer-heat, dampness, dryness and heat (fire) are six kinds of natural climatic factors known as "six qi". Human beings living in the natural world constantly contact with these natural factors. Under normal condition, the human body can adapt to the changes of climate which are indispensable to the existence of human beings. If the harmonious relationship between human beings and nature is broken, the body is unable to adapt itself to the changes of the climate, leading to the occurrence of disease. Under such condition, the six natural climatic factors become pathogenic factors.

The six climatic factors are characterized by the following features in causing disease:

- The cause of disease by the six climatic factors is usually related to seasonal changes of living conditions.

- The six climatic factors may singly or collectively attack people. For example, pathogenic wind may combine with cold, dampness, dryness and heat to attack people and lead to wind-cold syndrome, wind-dampness syndrome, wind-dryness syndrome and wind-heat syndrome.

- The nature of the diseases caused by the six climatic factors may be the same as or different from that of the six climatic factors. For example, invasion of pathogenic cold may deepen internally to transform into heat and so do accumulation of pathogenic dampness. Sometimes the nature of the disease caused by various pathogenic factors may vary due to the differences in constitution, which is called "secondary transformation". For example, frequent abundance of yang or frequent deficiency of yin may transform into heat after the invasion of exogenous pathogenic factors; frequent abundance of yin or frequent deficiency of yang may transform into cold after invasion of exogenous pathogenic factors; frequent abundance of dampness or deficiency of the spleen may lead to transformation of dampness, etc.

- The six climatic factors usually invade people from the skin into the muscles or from the mouth and nose into the lung and the defensive qi. That is why external syndromes tend to appear at the early stage of disease caused by the six climatic factors and gradually transmit to the internal.

Besides, clinically there are some diseases due to dysfunction of the viscera that appear similar to the pathological changes caused by pathogenic wind, pathogenic cold, pathogenic dampness, pathogenic dryness and pathogenic heat (fire), known as "five endogenous pathogenic factors", such as endogenous wind, endogenous cold, endogenous dampness, endogenous dryness and endogenous heat (fire) which are not directly caused by, but can result from, the six exogenous climatic factors. For example, attack by exogenous pathogenic wind can stir the endogenous pathogenic wind and exogenous pathogenic dampness can induce endogenous pathogenic dampness.

Wind

Wind is the main climatic factor in spring. That is why wind tends to cause disease in spring. But in other seasons wind also can cause disease. Wind is characterized by the following features:

1. Wind tends to float: Wind is a pathogenic factor of yang nature, characterized by floating and dispersion because of lightness. That is why wind attacks the upper part (the head and face) and skin first when it invades the body. So the disease caused by wind mainly involves the surface of the body, the head and the face with the manifestations of headache, running nose, sweating and aversion to cold, etc.

2. Wind tends to move: Wind is mobile and the disease caused by it is also changing (such as migratory pain of limbs in wind-bi syndrome), tremor of the limbs (such as

convulsion, spasm due to some special pathogenic factors of wind) and dizziness (such as subjective feeling of shaking or faintness or like sitting in a boat or car). Dizziness is usually caused by dysfunction of the viscera complicated by liver-wind. Exogenous pathogenic wind is often the factor that induces endogenous wind.

3. Wind tends to change: So the disease caused by wind is often characterized by sudden onset, immediate transmission and change as well as fast healing. For example, rubella is marked by quick fluctuation of cutaneous pruritus without a fixed location.

4. Wind tends to be complicated by other pathogenic factors: Since it is easier for wind to attack the body, other factors in the six exogenous factors often attach themselves to wind when they invade the body, frequently leading to exogenous wind-cold syndrome, exogenous wind-heat syndrome, exogenous wind-dampness syndrome and exogenous wind-dryness syndrome. That is why TCM holds that "wind is the leading cause of all diseases".

Cold

Cold is the dominant climatic factor in winter. So cold diseases, though may encounter in other seasons, are usually emerged in winter. The invasion of cold into the body is commonly due to cold weather and lack of cold control measures. Sometimes it is due to drench, walking in water and exposure to wind when sweating.

The invasion of wind is either superficial or internal. The former refers to external cold syndrome caused by cold attacking the surface of the body and stagnates the defensive qi while the latter refers to direct attacks of internal of the body and impairs the visceral yang-qi.

The following is a brief description of the nature of pathogenic cold and its characteristics in causing diseases:

1. Cold tends to impair yang: Cold pertains to yin and tends to impair yang. When cold attacks the surface of the body, it will impair yang in the superficies; when it attacks the internal of the body, it will impair the visceral yang. If yang-qi is impaired and cannot warm and transform qi, it will lead to cold syndrome due to functional decline. If cold impairs the superficies, the defensive qi will be stagnated, leading to aversion to cold and anhidrosis; if cold directly invades the spleen and the stomach, the spleen-yang will be impaired, leading to cold pain in the stomach and abdomen, vomiting and diarrhea; if cold directly attacks shaoyin, it will impair heart-yang and the kidney-yang, leading to aversion to cold, lying with the knees drawn up, dispiritedness, cold hands and feet, diarrhea with undigested food, profuse and clear urine, thin and indistinct pulse.

2. Cold tends to coagulate: Qi, blood and body fluid flow continuously inside the body because they are constantly warmed and propelled by yang-qi. If the pathogenic cold obstructs yang-qi, then qi, blood and body fluid cannot flow freely and will coagulate in

the vessels, bringing pain. If cold attacks the viscera, the visceral qi and blood will be stagnated, causing abdominal pain; if cold attacks the muscles and joints, qi and blood in the muscles and joints will coagulate, resulting in pain in the muscles and joints.

3. Cold tends to contract: Cold pertains to yin and tends to restrain the activity of qi, leading to contracture of muscles, tendons and vessels. If cold attacks the superficies, the muscular interstices will be stagnated, the muscles will be contracted and the defensive qi cannot disperse, leading to aversion to cold, anhidrosis and papules; if cold invades the limbs and joints, the tendons and vessels will become contracted, bringing on somatic pain, headache and spasm of the limbs.

Summer Heat

Summer-heat is transformed from heat and fire in summer. Summer-heat pertains to yang and usually appears after summer solstice and before autumn solstice. The attack by summer-heat is either due to hot weather or due to low adaptability of the body to the environment.

Summer heat is characterized by the following features:

1. Summer-heat is hot: Summer-heat pertains to yang and is hot in nature. So the disease caused by summer-heat is usually marked by a series of yang symptoms such as high fever, dysphoria, reddish complexion, thirst with preference for cold drink and full and large pulse, etc.

2. Summer-heat tends to disperse: Summer-heat pertains to yang and tends to disperse and elevate. Summer-heat disturbs the mind when it elevates, leading to dysphoria and dizziness or even sudden coma and unconsciousness in severe cases. Summer-heat induces sweating and consumes body fluid when it disperses, leading to thirst with preference for drinking water and reddish ancl scanty urine. If there is profuse sweating, qi will get lost, eventually bringing on shortness of breath and lassitude due to qi deficiency.

3. Summer-heat is often complicated by dampness: In hot season, heat fumigates dampness. That is why dampness is exuberant in summer and often mixes up with heat to attack people. Thus disease caused by summer-heat-dampness is often, apart from fever and extreme thirst, characterized by lassitude of the four limbs, chest oppression, vomiting and unsmooth loose stool, etc.

Dampness

Dampness is predominant in late summer but also can be encountered in other seasons. Since it is hot in late summer, dampness permeates everywhere due to fumigation and frequently causes disease. Sometimes drench or living in damp area also results in disease of dampness.

The following is a brief description about the nature and characteristics of dampness in causing disease:

1. Dampness is heavy and turbid: Dampness pertains to yin, so it is heavy. The attack by dampness will lead to symptoms as heaviness of the body or the four limbs, heaviness of the head like being bound, or heaviness and lassitude of the whole body. Dampness is similar to water and it often mixes up with water. That is why it is turbid. Invasion of dampness into the body often brings on the symptoms of turbid secreta and excreta, dirty complexion, excessive secretion of gum in the eyes, loose stool, mucous and bloody dysentery, turbid urine, leukorrhea and oozing eczema.

2. Dampness tends to block qi: Dampness moves slowly because it is heavy. So it tends to retain in the viscera and meridians, inhibits the flow of qi and disturbs the activity of qi, frequently leading to chest oppression and fullness, scanty and unsmooth urination and inhibited defecation. On the other hand, dampness pertains to yin and tends to impair yang-qi. Thus prolonged blockage of qi by dampness will prevent yang-qi from flowing, often causing exuberance of dampness and decline of yang. Since dampness pertains to earth in the five elements and is related to the spleen, it tends to impair the spleen, bringing on encumbrance of the spleen by dampness and stagnation of qi in the middle energizer. If dampness impairs yang, it will inactivate spleen-yang and further accumulate water and dampness, leading to diarrhea, scanty urine, edema and ascites.

3. Dampness is sticky and stagnant: These characteristics of dampness usually affect people in two ways. One is that the disease caused by dampness is not brisk. For example, the secreta and excreta are too sticky to be excreted. The second is that the disease caused by dampness is obstinate and recurring with long duration, such as damp-bi syndrome (damp-blockage syndrome), eczema and damp-warm syndrome.

4. Characteristic of dampness being descending and apt fixed to attack yin locations: Dampness is similar to water and characteristic of descending and apt to attack the lower part of the body. For example, edema caused by fluid-dampness is usually seen in the legs; vaginal discharge, turbid urine, diarrhea, dysentery and cankerous legs and mostly caused by down-pour of dampness.

Dryness

Dryness is predominant in autumn. So disease caused by dryness mostly appears in autumn. In late summer dampness permeates. But in autumn dampness disappears and the weather becomes cool and dry. Dryness can be divided into warm-dryness and cool-dryness due to difference in weather. The disease occurring at the early stage of autumn is a kind of warm-dryness because there is still some remaining summer-heat; the disease occurring at the late stage of autumn is a kind of cool-dryness syndrome because the weather is already cold in late autumn.

The following is a brief description of the nature and characteristics of dryness in causing disease:

• Characteristic of dryness being dry and puckery and apt to impair fluids: When invading the body, it is most apt to impair fluids, resulting in various xerotic symptoms such as dry mouth, nose and throat or even chaps, lusterless hair, dry stools and scanty urine and so on.

• Dryness likely to injure lung: As a tender viscus, the lung governs qi and respiration. It opens into the nose and is externally connected with skin and hair. The lungs are fond of clarity and moist and averse to dryness. Dryness pathogen frequently invades the human body through the mouth and nose and attacks the lungs, causing dry cough, scanty or sticky phlegm, gasping pain in the chest; when it damages the lung vessels, there is bloody sputum. The lung and large intestine are in exterior and interior relationship, so the failure of lung qi to disperse and descend and exhaustion of body fluids will result in lack of moistening of the large intestine and its dysfunction to transport, manifested as dry stools.

Heat (Fire)

Heat(fire) is the predominant climatic factor in summer. So disease due to pathogenic heat (fire) usually occurs in summer. However it can also be encountered in other seasons. Since there are two ways to describe the order of pathogenic factors in Huangdi Neijing, namely "wind, cold, summer-heat, dampness, dryness and heat" and "wind, cold, summer-heat, dampness, dryness and fire", so "fire" and "heat are often mentioned in the same breath. If we make a comparison between the fire and the heat, we can say that the heat is the manifestation of the fire and the fire is the nature of the heat. They are, to a certain degree, different from each other but intrinsically related to each other.

The following is a brief description of the nature and the characteristics of heat (fire) in causing disease:

• Heat (fire) tends to flame up: Heat (fire) pertains to yang and tends to flame up. So the disease caused by the pathogenic heat (fire) is marked by high fever, aversion to heat, extreme thirst, sweating and full pulse. When the pathogenic heat (fire) attacks the body, it may disturb the mind, leading to dysphoria, insomnia, mania, coma and delirium, etc. Since the pathogenic heat is responsible for irritability and rapid movement, the disease caused by it is characterized by acute onset and rapid transmission.

• Heat (fire) tends to consume qi and impair body fluid: Heat (fire) pertains to yang and tends to consume yin-fluid. If there is superabundant heat, it will drive body fluid out of the body in the form of sweat. So the disease caused by the pathogenic heat, apart from the manifestations of heat, is often accompanied by thirst with preference for drinking water, dry throat and tongue, dark and scanty urine and retention of dry feces due to consumption and impairment of body fluid.

• Heat (fire) tends to cause convulsion and bleeding: Convulsion means that when fire-heat invades the body, it burns and scorches liver meridians, exhausts fluids, causes the loss of nourishment of tendons and muscles, resulting in the syndrome of liver wind stirring up internally. So it is also called "extreme heat causing wind", clinically manifested as high fever, coma, spasm of limbs, upward squint of the eyes and opisthotonus etc.

Bleeding means that when fire enters blood vessels, it accelerates blood flow and burns the vessels, causing abnormal flow of blood, manifested as various bleeding, such as hemoptysis, epistaxis, hematochezia and hematuria, echymosis, excessive menstruation, metrorrhagia and metrostaxis etc.

• Heat (fire) tends to cause sores and abscesses: Fire invade xuefen, stagnates in local areas, causing erosion of muscles and pus, which are termed as sores, ulcers or abscesses. Clinically, it marked by are redness, swollen, burning and painful sensation in the local areas.

Pestilence

Pestilence is a kind of strong infectious pathogenic factor, quite similar to the pathogenic heat(fire) in the six pathogenic climatic factors in nature, but more serious than the pathogenic heat in toxicity. The diseases caused by pestilence are marked by acute onset, severe pathological condition, similar symptoms, strong infection and easiness to spread. Historical records show that diseases caused by pestilence often spread the disease far and wide with high mortality.

The commonly encountered diseases caused by pestilence are facial erysipelas, mumps, pestilent dysentery, diphtheria, scarlet fever, smallpox, cholera and plague.

Five Endogenous Pathogenic Factors

The so-called five endogenous pathogenic factors are endogenous wind, endogenous cold, endogenous dampness, endogenous dryness and endogenous heat (fire). Though they are called wind, cold, dampness, dryness and heat (fire), they are actually pathogenic factors due to dysfunction of the viscera. That is why the word "endogenous" is used to modify their names.

• Endogenous wind: Endogenous wind is produced by the liver, so it is usually called "liver-wind" and "internal disturbance of liver-wind". There are four factors responsible for the occurrence of endogenous wind. The first is extreme heat producing wind, referring to the disease marked by convulsion due to exuberant heat that scorches liver-yin and deprives the tendons of nourishment; the second is transformation of liver-yang into wind, referring to the disease marked by dizziness and infantile convulsion resulting from hyperactivity of yang transforming into wind and disturbing the upper orifices; the third is yin-deficiency stirring wind, referring to the disease marked by infantile convulsion and convulsion resulting from declination of liver-yin and inability of yang to hide that lead to failure of the yin-fluid to nourish the tendons; the fourth is blood-deficiency stirring wind, referring to the disease marked by muscular peristalsis and tremor resulting from failure of the deficient blood to nourish the liver and the tendons.

- Endogenous cold: The occurrence of endogenous cold is due to the deficiency of yang. The deficiency-cold of the viscera can be caused by either the deficiency of the kidney-yang or the spleen-yang or heart-yang. Since the kidney-yang is the source of yang-qi in the whole body, the deficiency of the kidney-yang is the predominant factor responsible for the occurrence of endogenous cold.

- Endogenous dampness: Endogenous dampness results from the spleen. Usually failure of water to transform due to dysfunction of the spleen may produce the endogenous dampness which encumbers the spleen and affects the transporting and transforming functions of the spleen or accumulates into phlegm and retention of fluid, further resulting in other diseases.

- Endogenous dryness: Endogenous dryness results from insufficiency of body fluid and is related to yin-deficiency. Since body fluid and blood can transform into each other, the deficiency of blood also causes dryness. The manifestations of endogenous dryness are often related to the intestines, the stomach, the lung and other orifices, such as dry nose, dry throat, dry eyes, scanty urine and retention of dry feces, etc.

- Endogenous heat(fire): The causes of endogenous heat (fire) are various, such as exogenous wind, exogenous cold, exogenous dampness and exogenous dryness that all can transform into heat; mental upset and extreme changes of emotions that often turn into fire; predomination of yang and deficiency of yin that usually produce the endogenous fire and heat; and excessive qi that frequently leads to fire, etc.

Healing Modalities in Chinese Medicine

TCM has a variety of natural healing methods that can help you resolve your health issues. These ancient healing forms have been used effectively—without harmful side effects—for thousands of years. These modalities reflect Chinese insight and ingenuity in creating methods that promote healing in specific ways.

Each and every TCM modality is based on Qi. You were born with a self-healing ability, and through the use of a particular healing form, TCM practitioners recharge that self-healing function in your body. These modalities can increase and balance your Qi, giving your body and being the healing support it needs to regain its healthy function.

Acupuncture

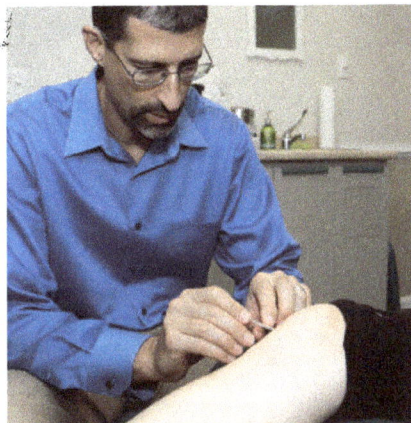

No one can really say how long acupuncture has been practiced. Ancient bone and stone "needles" thought to be thousands of years old have been found in modern excavation sites in China. What is known is that therapy with the technique of acupuncture has been helping heal people for ages.

It's impossible to define acupuncture without linking it to Qi, or energy. Everything in the Universe is comprised of energy. In your body, Qi flows through invisible energy pathways called "meridians," and it activates, warms, and nourishes your body.

Acupuncture needles—today, made of stainless steel—are used to relieve energy blockages at key acupoints along the meridians to help the Qi flow smoothly. An organ's function can also be readjusted by acupuncture to help restore internal balance and harmony among the organs.

It's also important to know that effective treatment is dependent to a great degree on the acupuncturist's skill and whether his or her energy frequency can match yours.

Pain, for instance, can come from different sources. It can be from an external cause, such as a sports injury, or from an internal condition, such as a Qi deficiency or Qi stagnation. Generally speaking, external conditions are easier to treat. Internal conditions tend to be more complex as the root cause is not so evident.

Is the key factor in acupuncture the needle, the acupoint, or the level of the practitioner? True acupuncture, also called "energy acupuncture," requires deep insight into what has caused the health problem and which organs have been affected. The needle is simply a vehicle between the practitioner's Qi and the patient's Qi. Bottom line, it's the understanding, skill, and energy level of the acupuncturist that makes acupuncture work, and not the needles or the selection of certain acupoints.

Acupressure

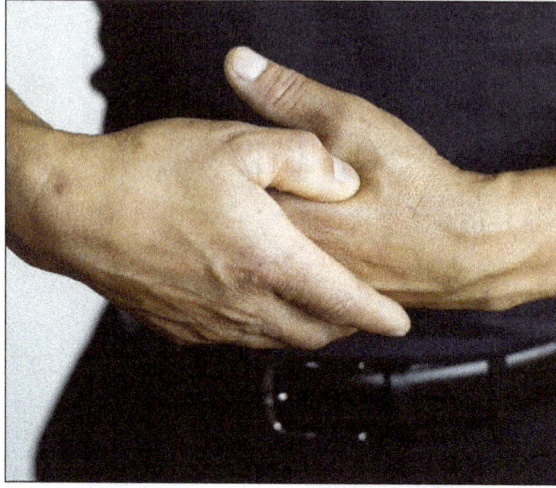

Authentic TCM acupressure, called tuina (twee nah) in China, uses specific hand techniques, or sometimes tools, to stimulate acupoints and meridians. With acupressure, Qi that is blocked or stagnant can be released and allowed to flow freely once again.

Though different than acupuncture, acupressure can be just as effective. Actually, for some conditions, like sports injuries and simple sprains, it's more useful and easier on the person receiving treatment. Sometimes, when it is appropriate, TCM doctors use acupuncture and acupressure in combination, which can accelerate the healing benefits.

Classical Herbal Therapy

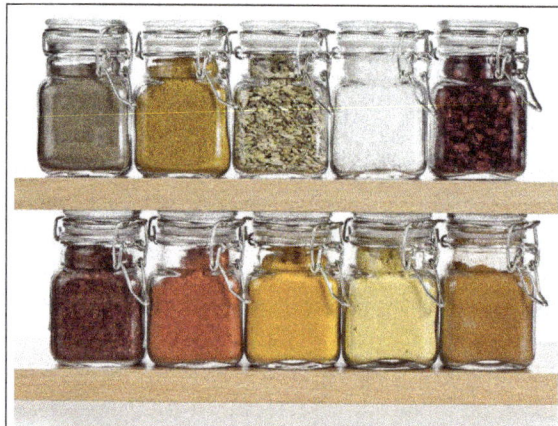

TCM has relied on herbal therapy as a healing tool for thousands of years. Along the way, it has identified and classified the essential properties of literally thousands of herbs and just how they act on the body-mind-spirit. Interestingly, an extremely wide range of objects fall into the category of TCM herbs: dirt, stones, bones, insects, a diverse selection of animal parts, as well as more common plant parts, such as leaves, blossoms, stems, and roots. TCM recognizes that everything is energy, and so unique energies that can impact the human body and energy system are not limited to the plant kingdom.

This holistic healing system uses herbs in a truly unique way: in combination. In a TCM formula the individual herbs used combine to make a substance that is much more powerful that the sum of the individual parts. In a formula the herbs act together as a team, with each herb performing a specific task within the body, to achieve the objective of the formula as a whole.

Eating for Healing

Food is something you eat every day—for most people, three times a day. If you stop and think about it, why not eat in a way that truly supports your health and well-being? This is precisely the approach TCM takes when it comes to food. TCM has understood the healing properties of food for millennia, and it knows the value of accumulating healing benefits from everyday actions, like eating, one day at a time.

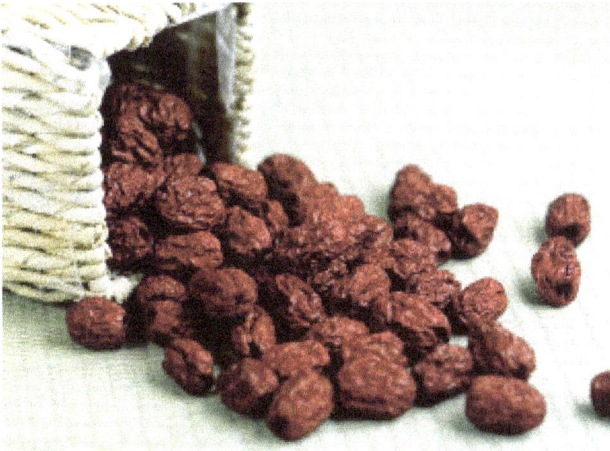

When TCM speaks about the value of food it is referring to qualities beyond physical characteristics such as calories, minerals, and nutritional content like carbohydrates and protein. TCM realizes that each and every food has a special essence—a healing essence—that works in the body at the energy level. Using the Five Element theory, which maps the interrelationships of all things, TCM practitioners prescribe foods that have an essence that heals particular organs that may be out of balance or in need of healing support. This is the essence of TCM's eating-for-healing approach.

TCM wisdom also teaches us to follow the seasons when selecting foods. This means regularly including foods in the diet that support the organ system at its peak during each season. Every season has a corresponding taste, according to the Five Element theory: for example, summer is associated with a bitter taste, fall with a pungent or spicy taste, winter's taste is salty, and in spring the taste is sour.

Qigong

The life force or energy that animates everything in the universe and your body is the very essence of Qigong. It's a Chinese practice that uses movements and postures and can create many physical healing benefits, but it's important to realize that Qigong is not physical exercise. It moves beyond the muscle and tissue and works in your body at the level of energy, or Qi.

Literally meaning "energy work," Qigong breaks down energy blockages and promotes the free flow of energy throughout your body's meridian system, the invisible pathways through which Qi moves and that connect everything in your body.

Consistent Qigong practice increases and balances your body's Qi. Working directly on your body's meridian system—your energy body—it stimulates and nourishes the internal organs, making the energetic communication between them more efficient. And by increasing the effectiveness of all body systems, Qigong helps conserve Qi. These qualities are important to your health because TCM theory says that in order to have good health you must have sufficient Qi that flows freely throughout your body and your internal organs must function together in harmony.

Five Element Psychology

If you speak with modern TCM practitioners, you will quickly discover that unbalanced emotions are the source of many modern health issues. How does TCM work with these kinds of health problems?

Chinese medicine looks deeply at the emotions as a gauge for health, yet it understands that a person's emotional state is not only a question of emotions but is also related to organ function. By adjusting the function of the organ (or organs) involved, there will be an accompanying adjustment in the emotions. You might wonder how this is possible.

In the TCM paradigm, your body is a whole, and your mind and emotions are completely connected. TCM understands that body, mind, emotions, and spirit are linked, and that an excess of any emotion can affect the function and balance of its corresponding organ. The reverse is also true: An imbalance in an organ's function can actually cause emotional issues.

Five Element psychology is based on TCM's Five Element theory, which is a comprehensive system that organizes everything, including your internal organs, into five Universal interacting groups or patterns. The Five Element theory perceives that each organ has a specific emotion related to it. The expression and level of any emotion therefore is closely tied to and dependent on the level of its corresponding organ's function:

- Liver is associated with Anger;

- Heart is associated with Joy;

- Spleen is associated with Worry;

- Lung is associated with Grief;

- Kidney is associated with Fear.

Benefits of Traditional Chinese Medicine

Traditional Chinese medicine is a type of holistic and natural medicinal system that has been in use for over two thousand years. It is designed to stimulate the healing mechanisms of the body, and can bring many health benefits to you both physically and psychologically.

Here are the health benefits of traditional Chinese medicine:

Reduce Inflammation

Reducing inflammation in your body is extremely important because inflammation serves as the root cause of a wide variety of different diseases, including heart disease, diabetes, autoimmune diseases, and even cancer.

Traditional Chinese medicine can help to reduce inflammation and the consequences associated with it through a number of different means, including herbal treatments, acupuncture, and acupressure.

In the process, Chinese medicine can also help you to stop any lifestyle habits that are harmful to your body and make inflammation worse, such as eating too much, smoking cigarettes, or drinking too much alcohol.

Improve your Muscle Strength and Flexibility

When we want to improve strength and flexibility in our muscles, we commonly turn to strength training exercises. That's great, but traditional Chinese medicine is another way you can improve your muscles as well.

In fact, practicing tai chi regularly provides you with an important aerobic workout, and practicing it for just three months can improve your balance, help you maintain or even enhance your flexibility and agility, and boost the overall strength in your muscles.

Protects and Improves your Cognitive Health

Protecting your physical health should be a top priority for you, but equally if not more important is to protect your mental health, and yet again traditional Chinese medicine is great for this.

Chinese herbs don't just help reduce inflammation; they can also help to relieve stress in the process. This is because Chinese herbs can effectively regulate the hormones that protect your brain, which also serves to control the immune response of your body. Using Chinese herbs decreases the risk of you developing dementia later in life as well.

Very Few Side Effects

Most medications and stimulants designed to help the body often come with a number of bad side effects, but fortunately, this is not the case with Chinese medicine. In fact, the few side effects that do come with Chinese medicine are practically harmless.

Improve the Quality of your Sleep

Last but not least, traditional Chinese medicine can help to improve the overall quality of your sleep. The typical adult needs an average of eight hours of high quality sleep each night, and getting this sleep helps improve blood circulation, calm anxiety, and improve your cognitive strength.

References

- Traditional-chinese-medicine-from-aqueous-extracts-to-therapeutic-formulae, plant-extracts, books: intechopen.com, Retrieved 29 June, 2019

- The-five-major-organ-systems, what-is-tcm: tcmworld.org, Retrieved 30 April, 2019

- Emotions-in-traditional-chinese-medicine: verywellmind.com, Retrieved 11 January, 2019

- Six-climatic-factors: tcmwiki.com, Retrieved 14 July, 2019

- Healing-modalities, what-is-tcm: tcmworld.org, Retrieved 18 April, 2019

- Top-5-health-benefits-traditional-chinese-medicine: sochealth.co.uk, Retrieved 7 May, 2019

Chapter 2

Model of the Body

The model of the body according to traditional Chinese medicine consists of numerous components such as qi, xue, jinye, zang fu and jing luo. The topics elaborated in this chapter will help in gaining a better perspective about these components as well as the relationships between essence, qi, blood and body fluids.

Qi

Qi (also known as chi) is usually translated as "vital life force," but qi goes beyond that simple translation. According to Classical Chinese Philosophy, qi is the force that makes up and binds together all things in the universe. It is paradoxically, both everything and nothing.

In Traditional Chinese Medicine (TCM), the concept of qi or chi has two main branches. There is the physical or nourishing portion of qi that makes up the air, water, and food that we take in. The other branch of chi is more insubstantial. It is the vital fluids and the energy itself that flows through our bodies.

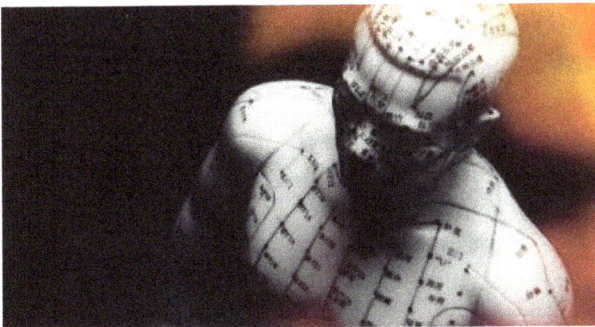

Chi flows along the meridian points of the body and
serves the basis for understanding acupuncture.

The first, as stated above, could be thought of as those things we take in and make a part of us while the second is what has already become part of us and is then released to continue the cycle of life. It is the imbalances and interruptions of this flowing force that is responsible for most human ailments whether physical, mental, or emotional.

Yin and Yang: To truly understand qi it is important to grasp the concept of Yin-Yang. Yin is that portion of qi that is cold, passive, solid, heavy, descending, moist and dark; it is the physical or brute side of the universe. Yang is ethereal. It is nebulous, hot, active, dry, rising and aggressive.

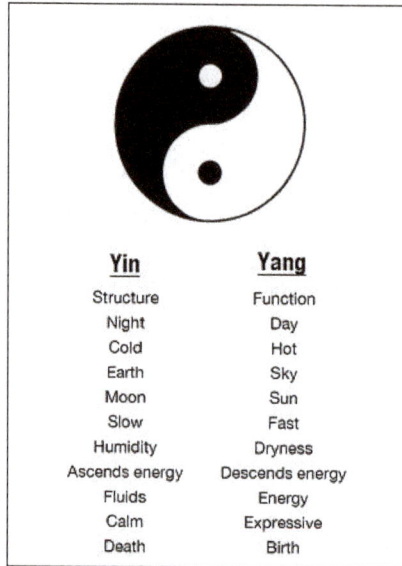

Yin	Yang
Structure	Function
Night	Day
Cold	Hot
Earth	Sky
Moon	Sun
Slow	Fast
Humidity	Dryness
Ascends energy	Descends energy
Fluids	Energy
Calm	Expressive
Death	Birth

A chart of different yin-yang relationships.

It must be understood that *yin* and *yang* do not exist outside of each other, but rather, that they reside within each other and must be kept in proper balance.

Form (yin) needs a function (*yang*); they are interdependent. It is this balance that defines and creates good health and emotions.

Maintaining Balance of Qi

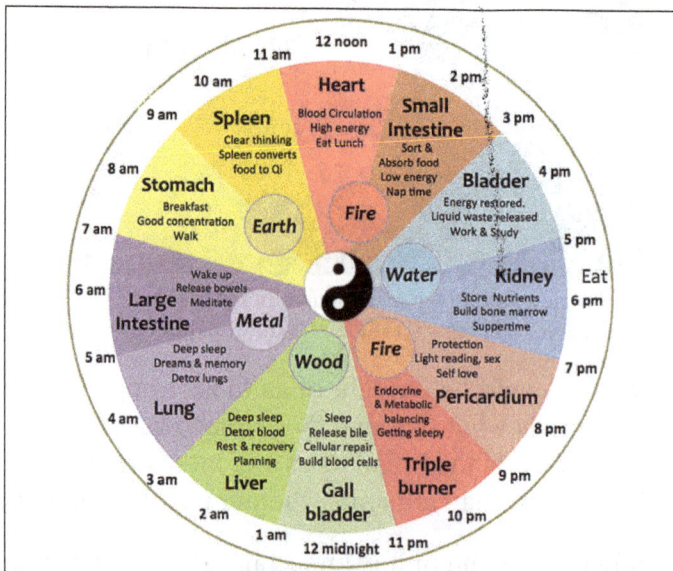

An advanced diagram showing the relationship between qi and the diurnal cycle.

As with yin-yang, qi needs to balance in order to maintain good health. If there is an imbalance of qi, illness can arise, with varying symptoms according to the type of qi and whether there is a deficiency or excess of qi. Curing the imbalance of qi is usually the main work of the different healing modalities in Traditional Chinese Medicine, such as acupuncture and tui na.

1. Qi Deficiency: In Chinese medicine, a qi deficiency can take many forms. It could be a lack of sleep, food shelter, clean water, fresh air or other physical things the body needs to function properly. It can also be a lack of sufficient mental stimulation, social interaction, and love.

2. Excess Qi: Excess qi can be as detrimental as a qi deficiency if not worse. It can arise as a result of environmental toxins, like polluted air or water. It can also arise from excessive physical activity, overeating, stress, or strong negative emotions.

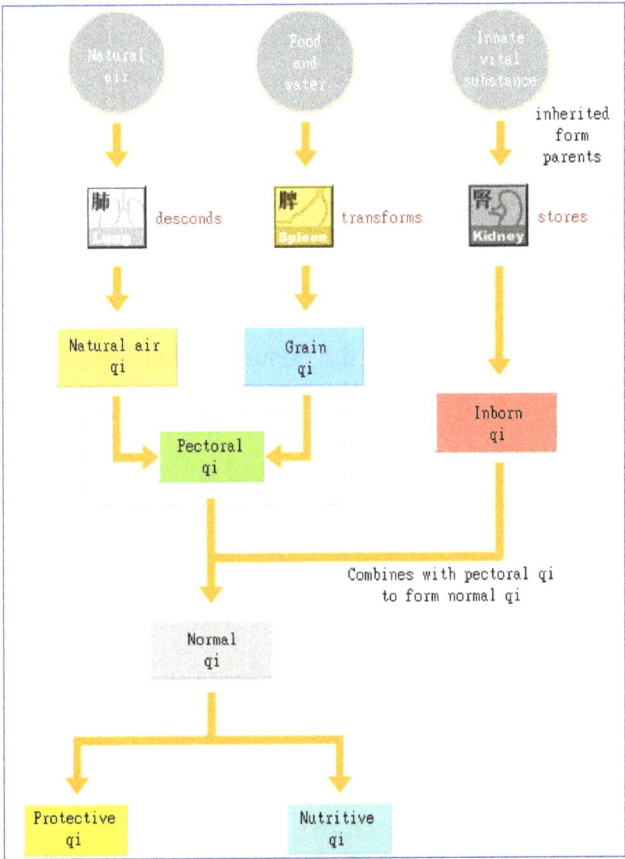

Qi flow chart

To avoid disharmony it is important to maintain a proper balance of all the different forms of qi that make up life. There are four types of qi within the human body:

- Parental Qi: Our parental or yuan qi is the qi that is inherited from our parents at conception. After conception occurs, parental qi is stored in the kidneys.

- Pectoral Qi: Pectoral or zong qi is qi that is produced by breathing. It is stored in the chest area.

- Nutritional Qi: Nutritional or ying qi is derived from eating foods and is responsible for the circulation nutrition throughout the body.

- Defensive Qi: Defensive or wei qi is responsible for protecting the body from illnesses. It is the yang of nutritional qi, meaning that it is also derived from eating foods, but serves a different purpose.

Functions of Qi: Each of the vital substances has Five Cardinal Functions: actuation, warming, defense, containment, and transformation. The five cardinal functions of qi are:

- Actuation: Qi is responsible for maintaining the vital life energy that is necessary for the body to grow and develop properly. This includes all the body's functions, such as the Zang-fu organs, meridians, and Xue (blood). If there is a qi deficiency, then the functional entities and vital substances will be negatively impacted, which can cause illness.

- Warming: Qi helps produce heat and regulates body temperature for normal functions to occur. A deficiency in qi can result in a lowered body temperature, cold limbs, and a disposition to hot drinks, as means to combat this.

- Defending: Qi defends the body against external elements, such as pathogens and environmental factors that can cause illness.

- Containment: Qi is responsible for ensuring that the body's organs and fluids kept in their proper places. In the case of xue, qi is responsible for regulating blood flow within the vessels and ensuring that they don't leak out. Qi also regulates Jinye (body fluids-sweat, saliva, etc.) and makes sure that only the proper amount is allowed to leave the body. Qi deficiency can result in symptoms related to body fluids and organ problems.

- Transformation: Qi is also responsible for transforming nutrition and air into different subsets of qi, such as blood.

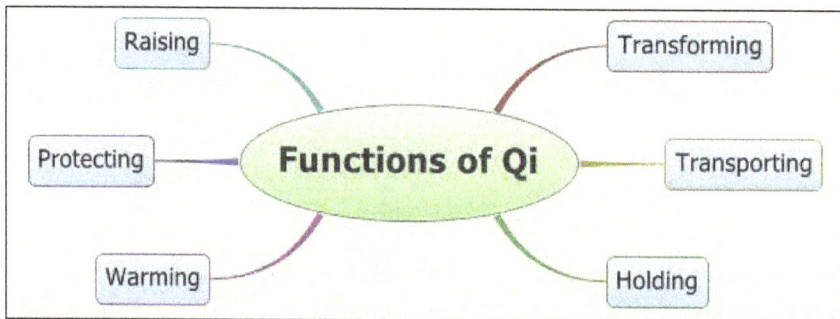

This chart is a summary of the qi functions. This groups holding and transporting together.

By now, it should be clear how important qi is in the human body.

Xue

Xue or blood which is mainiy composed of the nutrient qi and body fluid, circulates inside the vessels.

It is red in color and sticky in texture. Blood functions to nourish and moisten the body. It is vital to the maintenance of life.

Production of Blood

The basic substance for producing blood is essence, including the congenital essence (kidney-essence) and the acquired essence (food nutrients). The congenital essence is prerequisite to the production of blood. Only when the acquired essence has combined with the congenital essence can blood be produced. Thus deficiency of kidney-essence will make it difficult to produce blood. However, the congenital essence is already fixed after birth. In this case the acquired essence plays a key role in the production of blood. For this reason the functions of the spleen and stomach are key to the production of blood. If the spleen and the stomach are normal in functions, they can absorb sufficient food nutrients to produce blood. If the spleen and stomach are weak in absorbing food nutrients, the production of blood is inevitably reduced.

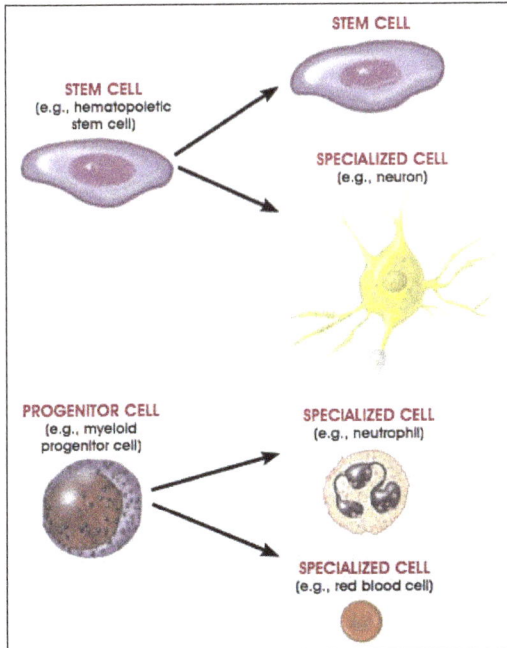

The transformation of the essence into blood is in fact a process of qi-transformation. The organs involved in such a process are the heart and the lung. The function of the heart in the process of blood production is called "reddening", because the heart pertains to fire in the five elements and red in the five colors. With the action of heart-fire blood becomes red. The lung participates in the production of the nutrient qi by inhaling fresh air from the outside. The nutrient qi is an important component of blood. So the functions of the lung directly influence the production of blood. Besides, the liver regulates qi activity and influences qi-transformation in the whole body with its dredging and dispersing functions, also exerting certain effect on the production of blood.

Physiological Functions of Blood

The physiological functions of blood are to nourish and moisten the body as described in Nanjing. Since blood contains the nutrient qi, it can nourish all the organs in the body. Through the meridians, blood transports nutrient substances to all parts of the body to nourish the five zang-organs, the six fu-organs, the five constituents, the five sensory organs and the nine orifices. It should be noted that blood is also the important material base for mental activities. If blood is sufficient, there will be sufficient vitality; if blood is deficient, there will be dispiritedness; if blood is in disturbance, there will be mental disorder. Since blood contains fluid, it can moisten the viscera and the body. When the fluid flows out of the vessels, it moistens the orifices and lubricate the joints.

Besides, blood also transports the turbid qi. When the turbid qi is transported to the lung, it is excreted from respiration. When it is transported to the kidney, it is discharged from urination. When it is transported to the superficies, it is excreted from sweating.

Circulation of Blood

The vessels in the whole body form a relatively close circulatory system for blood circulation. Such a system is known as blood vessels in TCM (Traditional Chinese Medicine) included in the concept of meridians and vessels. The minute capillaries are called blood collaterals.

Blood is propelled by the heart to circulate in the vessels. In fact the heart is the center of the blood circulatory system. In structure, the heart is connected with the vessels. That is why the heart can propel blood to circulate in the vessels. Since the circulation of blood is a circulatory process, the directions of blood circulation is either centrifugal or axopetal. The former means that the blood is propelled by heart-qi to flow out from the heart to the whole body through large vessels into large collaterals and fine capillaries. In such a way blood enters the internal organs to nourish and moisten the body. The latter means that blood accumulates from the fine capillaries to the large collaterals and the vessels into the heart under the propelling action of the heart.

Apart from the heart, other internal organs are also involved in the circulation of blood, including the lung, the spleen and the liver. Structurally the lung is connected with all the vessels in the body, known as "the lung facing all the vessels". With the association with the vessels, the lung distributes nutrient substances, like the pectoral qi, to the whole body and accumulates qi and blood from the whole body to assist the heart to propel blood circulation. The spleen commands blood, making the vessels compact, directing blood to circulate normally in the vessels and preventing it from flowing out of the vessels. The liver stores blood and regulates the volume of blood. Besides, the liver also governs dredging and dispersing, thus smoothing the activity of qi to promote blood circulation.

The factor that directly acts on blood circulation is qi. For example, heart-qi propels blood to circulate; lung-qi assists the heart to propel blood circulation; spleen-qi commands blood; and liver-qi regulates the circulation of blood by dredging and dispersing qi. If heart-qi is insufficient, blood will become too weak to circulate; if lung-qi is insufficient, there will be no opportunity for blood to disperse; if spleen-qi is insufficient, it will be difficult for the spleen to command blood; if liver-qi fails to dredge, it will lead to stagnation of qi and stasis of blood. Besides, visceral yang also plays an important role in the circulation of blood. For example, deficiency of yang will inevitably cause deficiency of qi, making it difficult for blood to circulate; deficiency of yin will bring on cold and exuberant cold will coagulate blood.

Other factors that may affect blood circulation are the state of the vessels and the changes of cold and heat. Generally speaking, phlegm, dampness, blood stasis, swelling and nodules can block or compress the vessels and obstruct blood circulation. Blood is characterized by preference for warmth and aversion to cold. So excessive cold slows down the circulation of blood or even causes blood stasis; excessive heat accelerates blood circulation and even leads to bleeding in severe cases.

Jinye

Jinye or body fluid Body fluid is a basic substance that makes up the body and maintains life activities. The main component of body fluid is water, also including nutrient substance. Body fluid is also a component of blood when it flows inside the vessels. However, body fluid also flows outside the vessels in the viscera and the body. If secreting or excreting from the five sensory organs and the nine orifices, body fluid becomes urine, sweating, tears, snivel, saliva and drool, etc.

Body fluid can be divided into two parts: thin fluid and thick fluid which are different from each other in property, location and functions. Generally speaking, thin fluid flows quickly and is distributed in the skin, muscles and orifices to moisten the related parts of the body. The thick fluid relatively flows slowly and is distributed in the viscera, cerebral marrow and joints to nourish the related parts of the body. Though different in texture and distribution, both the thin and thick fluids come from food and water transformed by the spleen and stomach, functionally flowing inside and outside the vessels to permeate and supplement each other. Physiologically they are not strictly separated from each other; pathologically "impairment of the thin fluid" is relatively light while "loss of the thick fluid" is relatively serious.

Production of Body Fluid

The digestive and absorbing functions of the stomach, the spleen and the large and small intestines play a key role in the production of body fluid. Body fluid comes from food, especially water and liquid diet. The production of body fluid comes through a series of physiological activities, including the functions of the stomach to receive and digest, the functions of the spleen to transport, transform and transmit, the functions of the small intestine to receive and digest, and the functions of the large intestine to transmit and change. Different viscera may exert different effect on the water taken into the body. So the metabolism of body fluid is accomplished under the coordination of different viscera.

Physiological Functions of Body Fluid

The physiological functions of body fluid includes the following three aspects:

1. Moistening and nourishing: Body fluid contains large quantity of water and nutrient substances to moisten and nourish the viscera and the body. To be specific, the thin fluid, distributed in the skin and orifices, mainly functions to moisten the body; the thick fluid, distributed in the viscera and cerebral marrow, mainly functions to nourish the body.

2. The transformation of blood: Body fluid not only flows outside the vessels, but also inside the vessels to participate in the production of blood. Blood is composed of two parts: body fluid and the nutrient qi. If body fluid is insufficient, the production of blood will be reduced, leading to blood deficiency.

3. The transportation of the turbid qi: Body fluid can hold various turbid qi and waste materials produced by qi-transformation and transport them to the concerned organs to be excreted out of the body through urination, sweating and respiration. The waste materials and the turbid qi are directly excreted in the form of fluid through urination and sweating. But the turbid qi excreted through respiration is transported to the lung first by body fluid and then exhaled out of the body. If body fluid is insufficient, the turbid qi cannot be quickly excreted out of the body, seriously affecting qi-transformation and causing various pathological changes.

Transportation and Metabolism of Body Fluid

The transportation and metabolism of body fluid are complicated, involving the physiological activities of several viscera. Body fluid, produced by the spleen and the stomach to absorb water and nutrients from food, is transported to the heart and the lung by the spleen to start its metabolic process. The viscera concerned with the metabolism of body fluid mainly include the spleen, the lung and the kidney as well as the heart, the liver, the bladder, the large intestine and the triple energizer.

The spleen, the lung and the kidney play a key role in the transportation and diistribution of body fluid. The spleen, governing transportation and transformation, transports body fluid to the heart and the lung; the lung, governing the regulation of water passage, transports body fluid to the whole body and down into the kidney; the kidney, governing water and separating the clear from the turbid, again transports body fluid that is steamed and qi-transformed during the formation of urine into the heart and the lung. In propelling the circulation of blood, the heart also promotes the flow of body fluid.

In this way body fluid is transported to the whole body to nourish the five zang-organs and the six fu-organs. After being used, the rest of water and the waste metabolic materials are excreted out of the body through certain routes. The excretion of body fluid involves the lung, the kidney, the bladder and the large intestine. Lung-qi, governing dispersion, depuration and descent, excretes the fluid from the skin and respiratory tract and excretes the fluid together with feces from the large intestine. Kidney-qi, governing water, transforms the fluid into urine to be excreted as urine from the bladder. Among these different routes, urination and sweating are the major ones for the excretion of the fluid. Only part of the fluid is excreted through defecation and respiration.

Besides, the liver and the triple energizer also play a certain role in the distribution and excretion of body fluid. Liver-qi, governing dredging and dispersing, promotes the flow and metabolism of body fluid by means of regulating the activity of qi; the triple energizer, serving as a water passage, directs body fluid to flow downward through it to the kidney. In the whole process of the flow and metabolism of body fluid, the triple energizer, connecting the upper with the lower, participates in the whole process of the production, distribution and excretion of body fluid. To be specific, the upper energizer participates in the distribution of body fluid as implied in the idea that "the upper energizer is like fog"; the middle energizer participates in the absorption of body fluid as implied in the idea that "the middle energizer is like maceration"; the lower energizer participates in the excretion of body fluid as implied in the idea that "the lower energizer is like a sewer".

On the whole, the flow and metabolism of body fluid involve several viscera, but the lung, the spleen and the kidney are the most important ones. So the dysfunction or hypofunction of these three organs will affect the flow and metabolism of body fluid, leading to phlegm, retention of fluid and edema.

Five Zang-organs Transforming Five Kinds of Liquids

The five kinds of liquids include sweat, snivel, tear, saliva and drool. TCM believes that these liquids are transformed by the five zang-organs.

The relationships between the five zang-organs and the five kinds of liquids are described this way: sweat is the liquid of the heart, snivel is the liquid of the lung, tear is the liquid of the liver, saliva is the liquid of the spleen and spittle is the liquid of the kidney.

1. Sweat comes from body fluid and is excreted out of the body through sweat pores under the steaming of yang-qi. The heart pertains to fire in the five elements. Heart-fire transforms into yang-qi to steam body fluid which comes out of the skin and becomes sweat. Thus sweat is regarded as the fluid of the heart. Insufficiency of heart-yang results in oligohidrosis while superabundance of heart fire brings on polyhidrosis.

2. Snivel refers to the nasal mucus that can moisten the nostrils. Since the nose is the orifice of the lung, so snivel is the liquid of the lung. If lung-qi fails to disperse, the nose will become stuffy and running; if lung-heat impairs body fluid, the nose will be dry with scanty snivel.

3. Tear comes from the eyes and can moisten the eyes. Since the eyes are the orifices of the liver, the tear is certainly the liquid of the liver. If there is wind-heat in the liver, the eyes will become tearing; if liver-yin is insufficient, the eyes will become dry because of scanty tear.

4. Saliva refers to the thin part of the fluid in the mouth. It can promote the intake of food. Since the mouth is the orifice of the spleen, saliva is the liquid of the spleen. If the spleen is weak, there will be profuse of saliva running out of the mouth; if spleen-yin is insufficient, the mouth will be dry because of scanty saliva in the mouth.

5. Drool refers to the thick part of the fluid in the mouth. Except with wetting and dissolution of food, making it easier to swallow, and the role of oral cleaning and protection, drool can nourish the Kidney-essence.

Zang Fu

Internal Organs are called Zang. These are the decision making and balancing centres of the body. They are the Heart, Liver, Spleen, Lung, Kidney and Pericardium. Their main functions are manufacturing and storing essential substances including Qi, Blood and Body Fluid.

External organs, or Fu are the Small Intestine, Gall Bladder, Stomach, Large Intestine, Urinary Bladder and Sanjiao. They receive and digest food, absorb nutrient substances and transmit and excrete wastes. They are allso called the hollow organs as they contain substances.

There are also extraordinary organs - the brain and uterus, which have no place in accumulating, filtering or circulating Qi but are supplied with nourishment by the body.

Each of the Zang is internally-externally connected to a Fu, and this pair corresponds to an element in the Sheng = nourishing cycle.

The pairs are as follows:

Internal	External
Heart	Small Intestine
Liver	Gall Bladder
Spleen	Stomach
Kidney	Urinary Bladder
Pericardium	Sanjiao

Correspondences

Five Elements	Zang	Fu	Sense Organ	Tissue	Emotion	Season	Environmental factor	Growth & Devel.	Colors	Taste	Orientation
Wood	Liver	Gall Bladder	Eye	Tendon	Anger	Spring	Wind	Germination	Green	Sour	East
Fire	Heart	Small Intestine	Tongue	Vessel	Joy	Summer	Heat	Growth	Red	Bitter	South
Earth	Spleen	Stomach	Mouth	Muscle	Meditation	Late summer	Dampness	Transformation	Yellow	Sweet	Middle
Metal	Lung	Large Intestine	Nose	Skin & Hair	Grief	Autumn	Dryness	Reaping	White	Pungent	West
Water	Kidney	Urinary Bladder	Ear	Bone	Fright & Fear	Winter	Cold	Storing	Black	Salty	North

Zang Organs

Heart

The channel of the Heart is connected to the Small Intestine. The Heart also opens into the tongue.

Functions of the Heart

1. Controlling blood and vessels: Vessels are the site of Blood containment and circulation, the impulse of the Heart sending blood incessantly through the vessels to nourish the whole body. When the Blood supply is sufficient the blood circulation normal, the complexion will be rosy and lustrous, and vitality full. The tissues and organs are well nourished and function properly.

2. Housing the Spirit: The Heart is considered the main organ is governing mental activities of the brain. Spirit, consciousness, memory, thinking and sleep are all dominated by the function of the Heart. According to Neijing: The Heart controls the vessels and the vessels supply the mind.

3. Opening into the tongue: The two functions of the Heart, ie, controlling Blood and vessels and housing the Mind, are closely related to the color, form, vitality and sense of taste of the tongue. This is also expressed as "the tongue is the mirror of the Heart".

Liver

The channel of the Liver connects with the Gall Bladder. The Liver opens into the eye. Its problems can manifest on both sides of the ribs, since the channels are bilateral.

Functions of the Liver

1. Storing Blood: The Liver possesses the function of storing Blood and regulating the volume of circulating Blood. During rest, part of the Blood remains in the Liver, while during vigorous activity Blood is released from the Liver to increase the volume of Blood in Circulation to the required amount. The Liver, therefore, along with the Heart, supplies the tissues and organs with Blood, and it influences menstruation as well.

2. Maintaining patency for the flow of Qi: This means that the Liver is responsible for harmonious and unobstructed functional activities of the human body, including the following three aspects.

- The Liver is related to emotional activities, especially depression and anger. Prolonged mental depression or a fit of anger may weaken the Liver so that is unable to promote the unrestrained and free flow of Qi. Conversely, dysfunction of the Liver is often accompanied by emotional changes such as mental depression and irascibility.

- The harmonious and free flowing functional activity of the Liver promotes the functioning of the other Zang-Fu organs, channels and collaterals, especially those of the Spleen and Stomach in digestion and absorption.

- This function of the Liver also affects bile secretion, its storage in the Gall Bladder and excretion into the intestines.

3. Controlling the tendons: The Yin and Blood of the Liver nourish the tendons, keeping them in a normal state of contraction and relaxation. When the Liver is supplied with ample Yin and Blood, the tendons are strong and free in extension and flexion.

4. Opening into the eye: Each Zang-Fu organ has a certain influence on the function of the eye. However, because the Liver stores blood and its channel directly communicates

with the eye, it has a closer relation to ocular function, such as vision and movement of the eye, than other Zang-Fu organs.

Spleen

The channel of the spleen connects with the stomach. It opens into the mouth. The main physiological functions of the Spleen are governing transportation and transformation, controlling the blood and domination the muscles.

Functions of the Spleen

1. Governing transportation and transformation: Transportation implies transmission. Transformation implies digestion and absorption. The spleen has the function of digesting food, absorbing its essential substances with a part of the fluid supplied, and transmitting them to the heart and the lung from where they are sent to nourish the whole body. Normal functioning of the spleen is required for good appetite, normal digestion and absorption, good nourishment and normal transmission of fluid.

2. Controlling blood: The spleen has the function of keeping the blood circulation inside the vessels and preventing it from extravasation.

3. Dominating the muscles: Normal function of the Spleen in transportation and transformation enables the muscles to receive adequate nourishment from the food essentials and thus maintains muscle thickness and strength.

4. Opening into the mouth: The spleen and the mouth co-ordinate functionally in receiving, transporting and transforming food. When the function of the Spleen is normal, the appetite will be good and the lips will be red and lustrous.

The Qi of the Spleen has the further function of holding and keeping the internal organs in their normal positions.

Lung

The channel of the Lung connects with the Large Intestine. The Lung opens into the nose.

Functions of the Lung

1. Dominating Qi and controlling respiration: The Lung is a respiratory organ. Through its function of dispersing and descending, it inhales clean Qi to supply the body's functions and exhales waste Qi. This is what is known as the function of "getting rid of the stale and taking in the fresh". As the function of the Lung greatly influences the functional activity of the whole body, the Lung is said to dominate the Qi of the entire body.

2. Regulating water passages: The dispersing and descending function of the Lung regulates water passages, promoting water metabolism. Its dispersing function turns a part of the body fluid into sweat to be excreted, while its descending function continuously sends a part of the body fluid down to the Kidney and on to the Urinary Bladder to be excreted as urine.

3. Dominating the skin and hair: Here the skin and hair signify the entire body surface. The Lung disperses the essentials of food to the body surface, giving lustre to the skin, gloss and luxuriance to the hair, and regulating the opening and closing of the pores.

4. Opening into the nose: The nose is the "gateway" of respiration. Unobstructed breathing and a keen sense of smell depend on good function of the Lung.

Kidney

The Kidney channel connects with the Urinary Bladder. It opens into the ear. Its main physiological functions are: storing essential substances and dominating human reproduction, growth and development, producing marrow which collects in the head forming the brain, dominating the bones and manufacturing blood, dominating body fluid and receiving Qi.

Functions of the Kidney

1. Storing essence and dominating reproduction, growth and development. The essence in the Kidney, also referred to as the Yin of the Kidney, consists of two parts:

- Ancestral essence inherited from the parents.

- Acquired essence transformed from the essential substances of food.

The vital essence of the Kidney is an important aspect of the Qi (vital functions) of the Kidney, greatly influencing the function of the Kidney in reproduction, growth and development. Neijing: "At the age of 14 for women and 16 for men, the Qi of the Kidney flourishes. Women will have the onset of menstruation, and men mill have seminal emission, both signifying the power of reproduction. When women reach the age of 28 and men around 32, the Qi of the Kidney is at its height, the body grows and develops, reaching the prime of life. When women reach the age of 49 and men around 64, the Qi of the Kidney starts to decline, the body begins to wither and at the same time the function of reproduction gradually fails".

2. Producing marrow, forming up the brain, dominating the bones and manufacturing blood. The Kidney stores essence which can produce marrow including spinal cord and bone marrow. The upper part of the spinal cord connects with the brain, while the bone marrow nourishes the bones and manufactures blood. The supply to the brain, the solidity of the bone, and the adequacy of the blood are therefore all closely related to the condition of the essence of the Kidney.

3. Dominating water metabolism: The part of fluid sent down by the descending function of the Lung reaches the Kidney. There is divided by the Yang function of the Kidney into two parts; clear and turbid. The clear - useful fluid it retained, and the turbid = waste fluid flows into the Urinary Bladder to form urine which is excreted.

4. Receiving Qi: Respiration is accomplished mainly by the Lung, but the Kidney helps through its function of controlling reception of Qi. The distribution of the clean Qi inhaled by the Lung to the whole body depends not only on the descending function of the Lung but also on the Kidney's function of reception and control.

5. Opening into the ear: The auditory function is dependent upon the nourishment from the Qi of the Kidney. Deafness in aged people is mainly due to deficiency of the Qi of the Kidney.

Pericardium

Its channel connects with the Sanjiao. Its main function is to protect the heart. The Pericardium is not generally regarded as an independent organ but as an attachment to the Heart.

Fu Organs

Small Intestines

The Small Intestine channel connects with the Heart, with which it is related. Its main function is to receive and temporarily store partially digested food in the stomach. Further digesting the food and absorbing the essential substance and a part of the water in food, the small intestine transfers the residues with a considerable amount of fluid to the Large Intestine.

Gall Bladder

The Gall Bladder channel connects with the Liver. Its main function is to store bile and continuously excrete it to the intestines to help digestion. This function of the Gall Bladder is closely related to the function of the Liver in promoting patency of vital energy. It is therefore said that the Liver and Gall Bladder preside over the unrestraint and patency of vital energy.

Stomach

The Stomach channel is connects with the Spleen. Its main function is to receive and decompose food. That is to say, the stomach receives and temporarily stores the food mass coming from the mouth through the esophagus while partially digesting it and then sending it downward to the Small Intestine. That is why the function of the stomach is normal when its Qi is descending and abnormal when its Qi is ascending. The

Stomach and Spleen act in co-operation and are the main organs carrying on the functions of digestion and absorption. It is said that the Spleen and Stomach are the source of health.

Large Intestine

The Large Intestine channel connects with the Lung. The main function of the Large Intestine is to receive the waste material sent down from the Small Intestine and, in the process of transporting it to the anus, absorb a part of its fluid content and then turn it into faeces to be excreted by the body.

Urinary Bladder

The Urinary Bladder channel connects with the Kidney. Its main function is the temporary storage of urine and its discharge from the body when a certain amount has accumulated. This function of the urinary bladder is accomplished with the assistance of the Qi of the Kidney.

Sanjiao

The channel of Sanjiao connects with the Pericardium. Sanjiao is not a substantial organ, but a generalisation of part of the functions of some of the Zang-Fu organs located in different sections of the body cavity. Sanjiao is divided into three parts:

1. Upper jiao (representing the chest) is a generalisation of the function of the Heart and Lung in transporting Qi and Blood to nourish various parts of the body. It is like an all pervading vapour.

2. Middle jiao (representing the epigastrium) is a generalisation of the function of the Spleen and Stomach in digestion and absorption. This may be compared to soaking things in water to cause decomposition and dissolution of substances.

3. Lower Jiao (representing the hypogastrium) is a generalisation of functions of the Kidney and Urinary Bladder in controlling water metabolism as well as storage and excretion of urine. It is like an aqueduct, a pathway for the flowing water.

Extraordinary Organs

Brain

Nei Jing: The Brain is a sea of marrow. Its upper part is under the scalp of the vertex, point Baihui = Du 20 and its lower part reaches point Fengfu = Du 16.

Yixue Yuanshi (Origin of Medical Sciences): "The sense organs, i.e., the ears, eyes, mouth and nose, are in the head close to the Brain. Owing to their highest and most obvious position, they may perceive objects, which will impress the Brain directly and remain in the Brain". Yilin Gaicuo (Medical Correction) suggested that thinking and memorisation are the main functions of the Brain.

As mentioned previously, the essence of the Kidney produces marrow that forms the Brain. The filling of the "sea" of marrow depends on the essence of the Kidney. Furthermore, the Heart, which houses the mind, and the Liver, which dominates the unrestraint and patency of vital functions, are also related to mental activities. A tenet of traditional Chinese medicine, therefore, is that mental activity is dominated by various organs, the Heart being the main one.

Uterus

The function of the Uterus is to preside over menstruation and nourish the fetus. Internal organs and channels related to the function of the uterus are as follows:

- Kidney: The Uterus is connected with the Kidney, and only when the essence of the Kidney is ample can the menstrual period recur regularly, and the impregnation and growth of the fetus be possible.

- Liver: The Liver performs the function of storing Blood and regulating the volume of circulating blood, which is also responsible for normal menstruation.

- Ren Channel and Chong Channel: Both originate in the Uterus. The Ren Channel regulates the function of all the Yin channels and nourishes the fetus. The Chong Channel has the function of regulating the Qi and Blood of the twelve regular channels. The Qi and Blood of the twelve regular channels pass into the Uterus through the two channels, affecting the amount of menstrual flow and its cycle.

Jing Luo

Jing luo, meridians or collaterals are the essential component parts of human body structure. The circulation of qi, blood and body fluid, the visceral functions as well as their correlations all depend on the transmitting and regulating functions of meridians to integrate the human body into an organic whole.

The theory of meridians, which is taken as an important component of the theoretical system of traditional Chinese medicine, concentrates on the study of the distributions, physiological functions, pathological changes of the meridians as well as their relationships with the viscera, body constituents, sense organs and orifices, qi, blood and body fluid.

Physicians in the past dynasties ceaselessly contributed their clinical experience to the supplement and enrichment of the theory of meridians since it formed in Huangdi Neijing. The theory of meridians supplementary to the theory of visceral manifestations, qi, blood and body fluid, has been the theoretical basis explaining the physiological activities and pathological changes of the human body and provides important guiding principles for clinical specialties, particularly for acupuncture, moxibustion, massage and Qigong.

Concept of Meridians

Meridian is a general term for meridians and collaterals. It serves as the pathway for the transportation of qi and blood throughout the body, thus connecting the viscera with extremities, the interior with the exterior as well as the upper with the lower. Meridians are the main trunks running longitudinally within the body, most of which run deeply inside and follow certain routes. Collaterals are the branches of meridians running reticular over the body. They run deeply or superficially within the body, most of which run in the shallow region and some often give a visible appearance on the surface of the body. The interconnection of meridians with collaterals throughout the body integrates the viscera, limbs and orifices, muscles and tendons into an organic whole, thus ensuring the normal performance of body activities.

Formation of the Theory of Meridians

1. Elicitation from the Pathological and Anatomical Knowledge: By the method of direct observation, ancient people gained a degree of knowledge about blood vessels, muscles and tendons, bones, viscera as well as the interrelationships between them, thus providing a basis for the formation of the theory of meridians.

2. Deduction of the Pathological Phenomena Over the Body: In clinical practice, it has been found that certain visceral disorders may be manifested on the corresponding superficial area of the body, where some pathological phenomena may occur, such as tenderness, nodes, rashes, and changes of luster.

When one viscus becomes diseased, pressing the corresponding superficial area of the body may relieve the pain inside. Hereby, it is inferred that there are special routes associating these acupoints, which serves as another basis for the formation of the theory.

3. Observation and deduction on induction and transmission phenomena of acupuncture and moxibustion: If the needles are accurately inserted into the right acupoints, the patient will feel a feeling of soreness, numbness, heaviness and distention, which is also called"needling sensation" or "Deqi" (arrival of qi) and may also transmit along certain routes to distant areas. When performing the technique of health preservation in Qigong, practitioners who concentrate their mind on Dantian point (the central area below the umbilicus), usually have a sense of qi flowing along certain routes. Such kind of sense and transmission is one important basis for the formation of the theory of meridians.

4. Summarization of the therapeutic effects of acupoints: When trying to summarize and analyze the main therapeutic effects of acupoints, ancient people found that acupoints with similar functions usually rank in the same route in a regular order. So it is presumed that the acupoints are connected with each other through some particular routes, which shows the great importance to the formation of the concept of meridians.

Composition of Meridians

The system of meridian is composed of meridians, collaterals and their subsidiary parts.

Main Meridians

Main meridians, being the trunk of meridian, may be classified into three categories: regular meridians, extra meridians and divergent meridians.

- Twelve regular meridians: Twelve regular meridians, also collectively termed as "the twelve main meridians", include three yin meridians of hand, three yin meridians of foot, three yang meridians of hand and three yang meridians of foot. These twelve meridians act as the main pathways in which qi and blood circulate throughout the body. They start and terminate at given sites, circulate along fixed routes, convergent in definite orders, distribute and flow with certain rules and are directly connected with certain viscera.

- Eight extra meridians: The eight extra meridians refer to eight important vessels different from the twelve main meridians, included the governor vessel, conception vessel, thoroughfare vessel, belt vessel, yin heel vessel, yang heel vessel, yin link vessel and yang link vessel. They perform the function of governing, connecting and regulating the twelve regular meridians.

- Twelve divergent meridians: The branches stemming from the twelve main meridians are referred to as the twelve divergent meridians, which respectively start from the limbs, run deep into the viscera, and emerge from the shallow regions on the neck. The divergent meridians of yang meridians separating from the meridians proper run inside the body arid return to the meridians proper while the divergent meridians of yin meridians separating from the yin meridians proper run inside the body and finally join the yang meridians to which they are interiorly and exteriorly related. The function of the twelve divergent meridians is to strengthen the connection between two meridians in interior and exterior relation.

Collaterals

The collaterals are the branches of the main meridians, including the connecting collaterals, superficial collaterals and tertiary collaterals.

- Fifteen connecting collaterals: The connecting collaterals are larger and major collaterals, which separate from the twelve meridians, as well as the governor and conception vessel respectively. Together with the large splenic collateral, they are so called "the fifteen main collaterals". The function of them is to strengthen the connection of the exteriorly-interiorly related meridians on the body surface.

- Superficial collaterals: The superficial collaterals are those running through the superficial area of the body.

- Tertiary collaterals: The tertiary collaterals refer to the smallest and thinnest branches of the whole body.

Subsidiary Parts of the Meridian System

The subsidiary parts of the meridian system refer to the parts that connect the twelve main meridians with the superficial and muscular portions of the body, including twelve muscle regions and cutaneous region:

- Muscles along twelve meridians: Muscles along twelve meridians, one of the subsidiary parts of the twelve main meridians, refer to a system where qi of the twelve main meridians "retains, accumulates, scatters and links"; in the muscles and joints, and serve to communicate the extremities with bones and control the movements of the joints.

- Twelve cutaneous regions: The twelve cutaneous regions are the twelve superficial areas of the body on which the functions of the twelve main meridians are reflected, and also the sites where qi of the twelve main meridians scatters.

Twelve Standard Meridians

Each meridian is a Yin-Yang pair, meaning each Yin organ is paired with its corresponding Yang organ.

- Yin (Arm) Meridians:

    ◦ Taiyin Lung Meridian of Hand.

    ◦ Shaoyin Heart Meridian of Hand.

    ◦ Jueyin Pericardium Meridian of Hand.

- Yang (Arm) Meridians:

    ◦ Shaoyang Sanjiao Meridian of Hand.

    ◦ Taiyang Small Intestine Meridian of Hand.

    ◦ Yangming Large Intestine Meridian of Hand.

- Yin (Leg) Meridians:
    - Taiyin Spleen Meridian of Foot.
    - Shaoyin Kidney Meridian of Foot.
    - Jueyin Liver Meridian of Foot.
- Yang (Leg) Meridians:
    - Shaoyang Gall Bladder Meridian of Foot.
    - Taiyang Bladder Meridian of Foot.
    - Yangming Stomach Meridian of Foot.

Eight Extra Meridians

The eight extraordinary meridians are different to the standard twelve organs meridians in that they are considered to be storage vessels or reservoirs of energy. They are not associated directly with Zang fu or internal organs:

- Conception Vessel (Ren Mai) (CV),
- Governor Vessel (Du Mai) (GV),
- Thoroughfare Vessel (Chong Mai),
- Belt Vessel (Dai Mai),
- Yin Link Vessel (Yin Wei Mai),
- Yang Link Vessel (Yang Wei Mai),
- Yin Heel Vessel (Yin Qiao Mai),
- Yang Heel Vessel (Yang Qiao Mai).

Circulation Rules of the Twelve Main Meridians

Circulation Directions

The twelve main meridians circulate in certain rules. Three yin meridians of hand run from the chest to the hand and converge on the ends of fingers with three yang meridians of hand in exterior and interior relation. Three yang meridians of hand ascend from the ends of fingers to the head where they connect with three yang meridians of foot. Three yang meridians of foot descend from the head to the ends of toes where they join three yin meridians of foot; three yin meridians of foot ascend from the toes to the abdomen and chest in which they meet three yin meridians of hand. The three yang meridians of both hand and foot all gather at the head and face, so it is said that "The head and face are the convergence of yang".

Convergence

Yin meridians and yang meridians in exterior and interior relation converge on the ends of four extremities. There are six pairs of yin meridians and yang meridians in exterior and interior relation, each pair converging on the ends of four extremities. The lung meridian of hand taiyin connects with the large intestine meridian of hand yangming at the end of the index finger; the Heart Meridian of Hand Shaoyin connects with the small intestine of hand yangming at the end of the little finger; the Pericardium meridian of Hand Jueyin connects with the shaoyang sanjiao meridian of hand at the end of the ring finger; the stomach meridian of foot yangming connects with the spleen meridian of foot taiyin at the great toe; the bladder meridian of foot taiyang connects with the kidney meridian of foot Shaoyin at the little toe; the gallbladder meridian of foot shaoyang connects with the liver meridian of foot jueyin at the hairy region of the great toe.

Yang meridians of hand or foot with the same name converge over the head and face. There are three pairs of yang meridians of hand or foot with the same name, each pair converging at the ends of four extremities. The large intestine meridian of hand yangming connects with the stomach meridian of foot yangming near the nosewing; ithe small intestine meridian of hand shaoyang connects with the bladder meridian of foot shaoyin at the inner canthus; the triple energizer meridian of hand shaoyang connects with the gallbladder meridian of foot shaoyang at the outer canthus.

Yin meridians of both hand and foot converge over the chest. There are three pairs of yin meridians hand or foot converging over the chest. The spleen meridian of foot taiyin connects with the heart meridian of hand shaoyin at the heart; the kidney meridian of foot shaoyin connects with the pericardium meridian of hand jueyin in the chest; the liver meridian of foot jueyin connects with the lung meridian of hand taiyin in the lung.

Distribution of the Twelve Main Meridians

The twelve main meridians distribute either inside the body or on the surface of the body.

Distribution Inside the Body

The distribution of the twelve main meridians inside the body is roughly longitudinal with each meridian curving and crossing in its circulation routes. There are intersections and convergences between the twelve main meridians, the twelve main meridians and their divergent branches, extra meridians as well as collaterals. Despite rare exceptions, intersection refers to the condition in which meridians usually run to the opposite side after crossing with another; convergence denotes the condition that meridians run in their original direction after crossing with another. In this way, there appears various complicated association between each component part of the body, which embodies the holism of TCM.

Distribution on the Surface of the Body

Distribution in the Four Limbs

The distribution rules of the twelve regular meridians in the four limbs are as follows: Generally three yin meridians are distributed along the medial aspect of the limbs and three yang meridians along the lateral aspect.

Each limb is distributed by Taiyin and Yangming meridians on the anterior border, Shaoyin and Taiyang meridians on the posterior border, and Jueyin and Shaoyang meridians on the midline. It should be borne in mind that in the lower limb, Taiyin meridian crosses and goes in front of Jueyin at 8 cun above the medial malleolus, therefore Jueyin is located in the anterior, Taiyin in the middle.

Distribution on the Head and Face

Yangming meridians of hand and foot run through the face and forehead, shaoyang meridians run through both sides of the head and taiyang meridians circulate through the cheek, forehead, vertex and occiput of the head.

Distribution in the Trunk

Three yang meridians of hand run through the scapular region and three yin meridians of hand emerge from the axilla. Of the three yang meridians of foot, yangming meridians run along the chest and abdomen (the front of the trunk), taiyang meridians along the back (the dorsal aspect), and shaoyang meridians along the sides. All the three yin meridians of foot run along the ventral aspect. The meridians running through the ventral aspect from the medial to the lateral are in turn named foot shaoyin, foot yangming, foot taiyin and foot jueyin.

As the twelve main meridians run symmetrically along both sides of the body in the chest, abdomen, head and face, back and four limbs, there are altogether twenty-four meridians.

Shen

Shen can be translated as "Spirit" or "Mind", and implies our consciousness, mental functions, mental health, vitality, and our "presence".

Shen lives in the Heart, where it retires to sleep during the night. If the Shen is disturbed, there may be insomnia. Shen is specifically said to live in the Blood Vessels (part of the system of the Heart) and to be nourished by the Blood. In TCM pathology, therefore, deficient Blood may fail to nourish the Shen. Alternatively, Heat (of various Organs) may disturb the Shen.

State of the Shen is said to be visible in the eyes. Healthy Shen produces bright, shining eyes, with vitality. Disturbed Shen produces dull eyes, which seem to have a curtain in front of them - as if no one were behind them. Often seen in those with long-term emotional problems or after serious shock (even a shock that occurred a long time ago.)

Healthy Shen depends on the strength of the Essence (stored in Kidneys) and Qi (produced by Spleen and Stomach). Thus, Shen is dependent on the Prenatal Jing and the Postnatal Jing. If Essence and Qi are healthy, the Shen will be nourished. As mentioned above, the Shen lives in the Blood Vessels, part of the Heart system in TCM. Blood is closely related to Qi in TCM, and is formed from the Postnatal Jing derived from food and fluids, hence Blood formation is simultaneous with that of the formation of Qi.

Jing, Qi and Shen are the "three treasures" in TCM. They represent three different states of condensation of Qi, ranging from Jing (more fluid, more material) to Qi, more rarefied, and Shen, more rarefied and immaterial.

This triad corresponds to the Heart, Stomach/Spleen, and Kidneys.		
Shen	Heart	Heaven
Qi	Stomach/spleen	Person
Jing	Kidneys	Earth

The Five Shen are the spirits associated with each of the body's five yin organ systems (Heart, Kidney, Spleen, Liver, and Lungs). The origin of the Five-Shen system is found within the Shangqing lineage of Taoist practice. Each of these spirits has a connection not only with a yin organ and its associated element, but also with the energy of a planet and a direction. To "wake up" the Shen of the organs is similar to "calling in the spirits" for a shamanic ritual. The Five Shen, when in balance, vibrate with a resonant beauty similar to the planets' "Harmony of the Spheres." Ultimately, within the context of our neidan (Inner Alchemy) practice, the Five Shen are returned to the unified Mind of Tao.

Shen: Emperor of the Heart

Within the Five Shen system we find something like a spiritual hierarchy: Shen—the spirit of the Heart—is the Emperor, with aspects of its power—like Ministers—residing as the spirits of the other organs. When these secondary spirits function as faithful emissaries of the Heart's Shen, communication between our organs is balanced and harmonious resulting in a happy well-functioning "Body Politic."

The element associated with the Heart's Shen is fire. Its direction is south, and the planetary energy that it embodies is that of Mars. As the emperor of the Five Shen, it is associated with the overall quality of our awareness, which can be perceived in the energy flowing through our eyes. Clear, sparkling, responsive eyes are one indication of healthy Shen—awareness that is vibrant, fluid, and intelligent.

Zhi: The Kidney's will to Act

The Shen of the kidney system is Zhi or will. Zhi is associated with the element of water, and it carries the energy of the direction north and the planet Mercury. Zhi is the minister in charge of the intention and effort required to accomplish things. This includes the effort and perseverance needed to succeed in our spiritual practice. According to Taoism, the highest use of personal will is to align ourselves with the "will of Heaven," i.e. with the Tao. The spirit-infused action arising from such a choice has the quality of wuwei: non-volitional and spontaneously skillful or "right" action.

Yi: Intellect of the Spleen

The spirit of the Spleen System is Yi or intellect. Yi is associated with the earth element. Its direction is center and its planetary energy is Saturn. Yi includes our capacity to use our conceptual mind to exercise discernment and to form intentions. An unbalanced Yi can manifest as discursiveness or unconscious internal chatter—a kind of over-thinking or "pensiveness" that damages the Spleen. A healthy Yi manifests as spirit-infused intelligence and understanding.

Po: The Corporeal Soul of the Lungs

The Po or corporeal soul is associated with the lungs and is the aspect of consciousness that dissolves with the elements of the body at the time of death. The Po belongs to the metal element, the direction west, and the planet Venus. Since the Po exists only within the context of a single lifetime, it tends to be associated with our immediate or more dense desires as opposed to the Hun, which expresses more long-range commitments.

Hun: The Ethereal Soul of the Liver

The Hun or ethereal soul is associated with the liver system and is the aspect of consciousness that continues to exist in more subtle realms even after the death of the body. The Hun is associated with the wood element, its direction is east, and its planetary energy is that of Jupiter. As our spiritual practice deepens, more and more of the Po–or physical–aspects of consciousness are transmuted or used as support for the Hun or more ethereal–aspects. As this process unfolds, we are, within our very bodies, manifesting "Heaven on Earth."

The Relationships among Essence, Qi, Blood and Body Fluid

Essence, qi, blood and body fluids are the basic material to form and sustain life activities of the human body. The metabolism including generation, distribution and discharge depends on viscera and meridians. Qi has the function of promotion and warming, while essence, blood, and body fluid have the function of nourishing and moistening, so qi pertains to yang, while essence, blood and body fluids pertains to yin according to the character of yin and yang.

Although they are different in nature, location, function, they are closely related and promote each other during physiological activities, and mutually affect and transmit in disease. Hence, they are closely related.

Relationship between Essence and Qi

Essence and Qi are closely related, so usually known as essential qi, such as essential qi in kidney, essential qi of food. Essence and qi are different in the yin-yang nature, i.e., essence pertains to yin while qi pertains to yang, and they can transform mutually.

Essence Generating Qi

Essence includes innate essence and acquired essence. Both combine and distribute to viscera to nourish qi of viscera and promote generation of qi. For example, essence stored in kidney can generate original qi, and food essence from food can generate nutritive qi. Therefore, essence can generate qi. Sufficient essence can generate sufficient qi to maintain vigorous functions of viscera; deficient essence can lead to deficient qi and hypofunction of viscera.

Qi Promoting Essence Generation

Essence generation depends on transforming function of viscera. For example, sufficient qi of the spleen and stomach means normal and active digestion and absorption, so that food can transform into essence needed by the human body. Therefore, qi's circulation is the promotive force for essence generation, i.e., sufficient qi ensures sufficient essence, while deficient qi leads to deficient essence.

Furthermore, qi can consolidate essence. For instance, kidney qi deficiency can lead to hypofunction of consolidation, manifesting as man's spermatorrhea and woman's diluted leucorrhea.

Relationship between Essence and Blood

Essence and blood both are generated from food, and supplemented by food essence. Both can promote and transform mutually, so it is said homogeny of blood and essence.

Essence Generating Blood

Essence is an important material basis for blood generation. Food essence transforms into blood through functions of the spleen, stomach, lung and heart, and kidney essence can generate marrow then to generate blood. Therefore, sufficient essence can generate sufficient blood. Either deficient food essence or kidney essence can lead to deficient blood generation manifesting as blood deficiency.

Blood Generating Essence

Essence of the human body is mainly stored in kidney. Kidney essence at first is inherited from parents and supplemented by acquired food essence. During the generation and distribution of kidney essence, blood is an important stage, for it can supplement kidney essence. For example, the liver stores blood, so that liver blood can nourish kidney essence. Therefore, sufficient blood can generate sufficient essence, while deficient blood can lead to deficient essence.

Relationship between Qi and Blood

Qi is active and pertains to yang while blood is static and pertains to yin. So the relationship between qi and blood can be understood according to the relationship between yin and yang. In TCM the relationship between qi and blood is generalized as "qi is the marshal of blood and blood is the mother of qi". Here "marshal" means governing and "mother" means source and foundation. Since qi pertains to yang, it can govern the circulation of blood; because blood pertains to yin, it is the source for qi-transformation. However, the relationship between qi and blood is not so simple as mentioned above.

Effect of Qi on Blood

The effect of qi on blood is mainly demonstrated in three aspects, i.e. qi producing blood, qi promoting the circulation of blood and qi controlling blood.

Qi Producing Blood

Qi promotes the production of blood in various ways. In terms of the composition, the nutrient qi is the main component of blood, indicating that the nutrient qi produces blood. In terms of the transformation of blood, the production of blood depends on qi-transformation. The material needed for the production of blood is the food nutrient transformed and absorbed by the spleen and the stomach. The normal functions of the spleen and the stomach are directly related to spleen-qi and stomach-qi. If spleen-qi and stomach-qi are vigorous, blood-producing function will be vigorous too. If spleen-qi and stomach-qi are deficient, blood-producing function will be weakened. In fact the transformation of the food nutrients into blood still needs the transformation of other visceral qi. For example, only when the food nutrients has combined with kidney-essence can the process of transforming the nutrients into blood be accomplished; only when blood transformed from the food nutrients and the kidney-essence has been processed by the transforming activity of heart-qi and lung-qi, especially heart-qi, can blood become red. If the functions of the spleen and the stomach are weak due to qi deficiency or if the transforming activity of visceral qi becomes weak, the normal process of blood transformation will be affected, leading to blood deficiency.

Qi Promoting the Circulation of Blood

Blood depends on the propelling function of qi to circulate. That is why TCM holds that "normal flow of qi ensures normal circulation of blood, stagnation of qi leads stasis of blood". In terms of visceral functions, heart-qi is the primary motivation of blood circulation; lung-qi assists the heart to propel blood to circulate; liver-qi promotes the circulation of blood. If qi is too weak to propel blood, blood will flow slowly; if qi activity is obstructed, blood will become stagnant; if qi activity is in disorder, blood will flow abnormally.

Qi Controlling Blood

Qi controlling blood means that qi directs blood to circulate inside the vessels and prevents it from flowing out of the vessels. The kind of qi that can control blood and direct it to flow inside the vessels is spleen-qi. That is why TCM holds that "the spleen commands blood". If qi fails to control blood due to deficiency, blood will flow out of the vessels, leading to bleeding.

Effect of Blood on Qi

The effect of blood on qi is demonstrated in two aspects: Carrying qi and producing qi.

Blood Carrying Qi

Blood pertains to yin and is static, so it keeps on flowing inside. Qi pertains to yang and is active, so it tends to move to the outside. When qi and blood have combined with each other, blood has acquired a motivation to move and qi has obtained a carrier to attach to. That is why it is said that blood can carry qi. That is to say that only when qi has attached itself to blood can it avoid dispersion and loss. Clinically massive hemorrhage is usually accompanied by loss of qi. Therapeutically, apart from using the therapy for supplementing blood and stopping hemorrhage, other therapeutic methods for supplementing qi and stopping prostration must be resorted.

Blood Producing Qi

Qi and blood, pertaining to yin and yang respectively, can transform into each other and produce each other. The primordial qi is produced by the congenital essence in the kidney and the food nutrients transformed by the spleen and the stomach. The normal functions of these organs all depend on nutrients provided by blood flowing in the vessels, and so do the other viscera and meridians. Thus the production of qi by blood is accomplished through its provision of nutrients for the viscera and meridians.

Relationship between Qi and Body Fluid

The relationship between qi and body fluid is similar to the relationship between qi and blood, because body fluid is a component of blood. Besides, body fluid exists not only in the vessels, but also in all the tissues and organs in the body. In this sense, the relationship between qi and body fluid differs in some way from the relationship between qi and blood.

Effect of Qi on Body Fluid

The effect of qi on body fluid is demonstrated in three aspects: qi producing body fluid, qi promoting the flow of body fluid and qi controlling body fluid.

Qi Producing Body Fluid

Body fluid comes from the water and nutrients of food transformed by the spleen and stomach. The spleen and stomach play an important role in the production of body fluid. If spleen-qi and stomach-qi are sufficient and if the digesting and absorbing functions are normal, the transformation and production of body fluid will be sufficient; if spleen-qi and stomach-qi are deficient and if the digesting and absorbing functions are abnormal, the transformation and production of body fluid will be reduced.

Qi Promoting the Flow of Body Fluid

The flow of body fluid, including the distribution and excretion, depends on the propelling function of qi. At the early stage body fluid is transported by spleen-qi to the heart and the lung; heart-qi propels body fluid and blood to flow; lung-qi disperses the fluid in the skin and viscera on the one hand, and descends the fluid to the kidney and the bladder on the other; the kidney and the bladder, through qi-transformation, transports the lucid part of the fluid to the heart and the lung on the one hand, and descends the turbid part of the fluid to transform it into urine to be discharged out of the body on the other. Since the flow and metabolism of body fluid all depend on the propelling and transforming functions of qi, the state of qi and the activity of qi directly affect the flow and metabolism of body fluid. If qi deficiency or qi stagnation occurs, the fluid will accumulate and turn into phlegm and edema. That is why it is said in TCM that "normal flow of qi ensures normal flow of water and stagnation of qi leads to stagnation of water."

Qi Controlling Body Fluid

Under the propelling and transforming action of qi, the metabolism of the body is demonstrated in two ways: opening and closing. Opening means to excrete the remaining part of fluid out of the body and closing means to keep certain amount of water needed in the body. The way that qi keeps body fluid in the body is called "qi controlling body fluid". The ways to excrete water from the body include urination and sweating. If qi fails to control body fluid due to deficiency, it will lead to abnormal urination and sweating, such as poliguria, incontinence of urine, enuresis and polyhidrosis, etc.

Effect of Body Fluid on Qi

The effect of body fluid on qi is demonstrated in two ways: Carrying qi and producing qi.

Body Fluid Carrying Qi

Body fluid is the carrier of qi and qi must attach itself to body fluid in order to flow to the whole body. This theory can be understood from two angles. On the one hand, blood produced by body fluid in the vessels can carry the nutrient qi; on the other hand, body fluid flowing in other tissues and organs can carry the defensive qi. If great quantity of body fluid is lost, qi will be exhausted accordingly. This state is called "loss of body fluid followed by exhaustion of qi". In severe cases, it will become "loss of body fluid followed by loss of qi".

Body Fluid Producing Qi

Body fluid, just like blood, can produce qi. On the one hand, body fluid inside the vessels transforms into blood to nourish the viscera so as to maintain sufficiency of qi in these viscera and the body.

Relationship between Blood and Body Fluids

The relationship between blood and body fluids can be generalized as homogeny of body fluids and blood. First, both are generated from food essence through spleen and stomach's digestion and absorption; also body fluids is consisting part of blood for body fluids generated by the spleen and stomach ascends to the heart and lung to become blood combined with nutrient qi. Second, body fluids and blood can mutually transform. Body fluids outside vessels can permeate into vessels to become a part of blood while body fluids consisting of blood can permeate out vessels to become body fluids. So, both depend on each other and mutually transform.

Pathologically blood and body fluids can inter-affect. For example, excessive bleeding can cause body fluids outside vessels to permeate into vessels to supplement blood volume. Hence, patients of excessive bleeding usually are with symptoms of dry mouth, dry throat, scanty urine,dry skin due to deficient body fluids. Excessive loss of body fluids can cause body fluids inside vessels to permeate outside vessels to supplement body fluids outside vessels, resulting into empty blood vessels or deficient body fluids and dry blood. Hence, patients of severe bleeding should avoid diaphoresis and diuresis; patients of severe body fluids loss such as severe sweating, vomiting, diarrhea, should avoid drugs or formulas to remove blood stasis, so as to avoid further damaging body fluids and blood, which are the clinical application of the theory homogeny of body fluids and blood sharing the same origin.

References

- Qi-in-traditional-chinese-medicine: amcollege.edu, Retrieved 21 July, 2019

- Zangfu, acupuncture: innerpath.com.au, Retrieved 13 July, 2019

- Jinye-body-fluids, wiki: tcmwiki.com, Retrieved 24 March , 2019

- Circulation-rules-of-the-twelve-main-meridians, meridians: tcmwiki.com, Retrieved 13 June, 2019

- Shen-spirit-chinese-medicine, get, foundations-chinese-medicine: sacredlotus.com, Retrieved 21 March , 2019

- Introduction-to-the-five-shen-3183169: learnreligions.com, Retrieved 12 April, 2019

- The-relationships-among-essence-qi-blood-and-body-fluid, wiki: tcmwiki.com, Retrieved 23 June, 2019

Chapter 3

Chinese Herbology

The branch of traditional Chinese medicine which makes use of plant elements as well as animal, human and mineral products for the treatment of ailments is termed as Chinese herbology. The diverse applications of Chinese herbology for the purpose of qi-regulation, heat clearing and phlegm resolution have been thoroughly discussed in this chapter.

Chinese herbology or Chinese materia medica, the Chinese art of combining medicinal herbs, is an important aspect of traditional Chinese medicine. Crude medicines (naturally occurring unrefined substances intended for medical use) and prepared drugs are used in combinations to treat patients according to traditional Chinese medical theory. Each herbal medicine prescription is a tailored to the individual patient and includes one or two main ingredients that target the illness, plus additional ingredients to adjust the formula to the particular patient's balance of yin/yang. Unlike in the production of Western medications, the balance and interaction of all the ingredients in a Chinese herbal prescription is considered more important than the effects of the individual ingredients. Chinese herbology incorporates ingredients from all parts of plants, including the roots, leaves, stems, flowers, and fruits, and also ingredients from animals and minerals.

The Divine Farmer's Herb-Root Classic, first compiled around 206 B.C.E. and attributed to Shennong, a legendary ruler of China who is believed to have taught ancient China the practices of agriculture, includes 365 medicines. During the Neo-Confucian Song-Jin-Yuan era (tenth to twelfth centuries), the theories of the Five Phases (Tastes) and the Twelve Channels (Meridians) were applied to herbology. The Compendium of Materia Medica (Ben Cao Gangmu) compiled during the Ming dynasty by Li Shizhen, is still used today for consultation and reference. It lists 1,892 distinct herbs, and about 11,096 prescriptions to treat common illnesses.

Chinese herbology is the Chinese art of combining medicinal herbs. Herbology is one of the more important aspects of traditional Chinese medicine (TCM). Each herbal medicine prescription is a cocktail of many herbs tailored to the individual patient and based on traditional Chinese medical theory. One batch of herbs is typically decocted twice over the course of one hour. The practitioner usually designs a remedy using one or two main ingredients that target the illness, then adds many additional ingredients to adjust the formula to the particular patient's yin/yang conditions. Sometimes, ingredients are needed to cancel out toxicity or side-effects of the main ingredients.

Some herbs require the use of other ingredients as catalysts, without which the brew is ineffective. A crucial element in traditional Chinese medicine is the treatment of each patient as an individual.

Chinese herbology often incorporates ingredients from all parts of plants, including the roots, leaves, stems, flowers, and fruits, and also ingredients from animals and minerals. The use of parts of endangered species (such as seahorses, rhinoceros horns, and tiger bones) has created controversy and resulted in a black market of poachers who hunt restricted animals. Many herbal manufacturers have discontinued the use of any parts from endangered animals.

Categorizing Chinese Herbs

Chinese physicians used several different methods to classify traditional Chinese herbs:

- The Four Natures
- The Five Tastes
- The Meridians

The earlier (Han through Tang eras) Ben Cao (Materia Medicae) began with a three-level categorization:

Low level—drastically acting, toxic substances; Middle level—herbs with medicinal physiological effects; High level—herbs for the enhancement of health and spirit.

During the Neo-Confucian Song-Jin-Yuan era (tenth to twelfth centuries), the theoretical framework of acupuncture theory, which was rooted in Han Confucian theory, was formally applied to herbal categorization, which had previously been the domain of Daoist natural science. In particular, the theories of the Five Phases (Tastes) and the Twelve Channels (Energy Meridians) came to be used after this period.

Four Natures

The Four Natures theory pertains to the degree of yin and yang, cold (extreme yin), cool, neutral, warm and hot (extreme yang). The patient's internal balance of yin and yang is taken into account when the herbs are selected. For example, medicinal herbs of "hot," yang nature are used when the person is suffering from internal cold that requires to be purged, or when the patient has a general cold constituency. Sometimes an ingredient is added to offset the extreme effect of one herb.

Five Tastes

The "five tastes" are pungent, sweet, sour, bitter and salty, each of which has its functions and characteristics. For example, pungent herbs are used to generate sweat and to direct and vitalize qi and the blood. Sweet-tasting herbs often tone or harmonize bodily systems. Some sweet-tasting herbs also exhibit a bland taste, which helps drain dampness through diuresis. Pungent herbs stimulate, warm, raise qi from the interior to the exterior. Sour taste most often is astringent and consolidates qi and secretions, while bitter herbs drain qi downward, dispel heat, purge the bowels and get rid of dampness by drying them out. Salty tastes soften hard masses as well as purge and open the bowels.

Pungent herbs strengthen the lungs and large intestine, sweet herbs harmonize the spleen and stomach, sour herbs nourish the liver and gallbladder, and bitter herbs strengthen the heart and small intestine.

Meridians

The Meridians refer to currents of energy which flow through different organs and parts of the body. Certain herbs are linked with specific meridians and therefore act upon the organs associated with them. For example, menthol is pungent, cool and is linked with the lungs and the liver. Since the lungs are the organ which protects the body from the invasion of colds and influenza, menthol can help purge invading heat toxins caused by hot "wind."

Chinese Patent Medicine

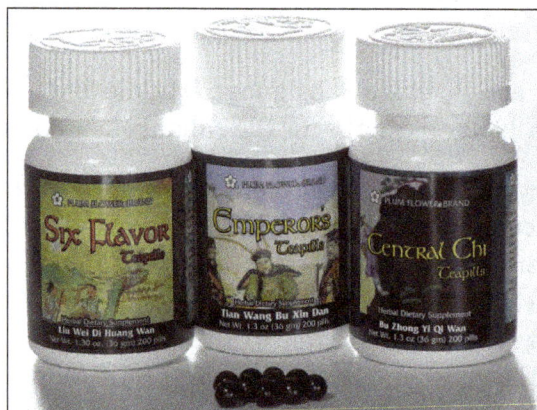

Characteristic little black pills of Chinese patent medicine.

Chinese patent medicine are standardized herbal formulas. Several herbs and other ingredients are dried and ground, then mixed into a powder and formed into pills. The binder is traditionally honey. The pills are characteristically small, round and black. Chinese patent medicines are easy and convenient, but are not easy to customize for a particular patient. They are best used when a patient's condition is not severe and the medicine can be taken as a long-term treatment.

These medicines are not "patented" in the traditional sense of the word. No one has exclusive rights to the formula. Instead, "patent" refers to the standardization of the formula. All Chinese patent medicines of the same name will have the same proportions of ingredients.

Chinese Herbal Therapy

Chinese Herbal Therapy is a major part of Traditional Chinese Medicine. It has been used for centuries in China, where herbs are considered fundamental therapy for many acute and chronic conditions.

Conditions Best Treated with Chinese Herbal Therapy

Like acupuncture, Chinese herbs can address unhealthy body patterns that manifest in a variety of symptoms and complaints. Chinese herbal therapy aims to help you regain homeostasis, or balance, in your body and to strengthen your body's resistance to disease. Chinese herbs may be used to:

- Decrease cold/flu symptoms,

- Increase your energy,

- Improve your breathing,

- Improve digestion,

- Improve your sleep,

- Decrease pain,

- Improve menopausal symptoms,

- Help regulate menstrual cycles if infertility is an issue.

Chinese herbal therapy can also be a valuable additional therapy following cancer treatment to aid the body's recovery from the after-effects of chemotherapy and radiation. Chinese herbs are useful in rehabilitation for other chronic diseases too. We may recommend Chinese herbal therapy when:

- You have multiple symptoms or they are hard to pinpoint.

- You've exhausted traditional medical options and nothing seems to help.

- You need therapy to counteract side effects of prescribed medication.

- You are interested in preventive treatment.

Traditional Chinese Herbal Remedies

Traditional Chinese herbal remedies are part of traditional Chinese medicine (TCM) and have been used in China for thousands of years. Traditional Chinese herbal remedies are a large part of TCM. They can be given as pills, teas, powders, liquid extracts or syrups. Hundreds of different types of herbs are used in TCM, and TCM practitioners often use combinations of herbs rather than a single herb.

Practitioners of traditional Chinese medicine often use herbal remedies along with other therapies, such as acupuncture, massage and tai chi.

Traditional Chinese Herbal Remedies as a Complementary Therapy

There is no evidence at this time that traditional Chinese herbal remedies can treat cancer itself. Many research studies have focused on TCM herbal remedies, but the research has only been reported in Chinese language journals. Many evidence-based organizations are concerned that the studies are not of high quality and that only positive results are published. So our current knowledge of traditional Chinese herbal remedies is limited.

Some research suggests that other TCM methods, such as acupuncture, tai chi and massage, may help people cope with the physical and emotional side effects of conventional cancer treatments.

Side Effects and Risks of Traditional Chinese Herbal Remedies

Talk to the healthcare team if you are thinking about taking any traditional Chinese herbal remedies. Let the TCM practitioner know about the cancer diagnosis and any conventional cancer treatments you are having.

Side effects of traditional Chinese herbal remedies will depend on the herbs and the combination of herbs in the preparation.

There have been cases of traditional Chinese herbal remedies containing prescription drugs that weren't listed on the label, which could cause serious side effects. Other herbs used in TCM have been found to be contaminated with toxic metals such as lead, mercury or arsenic.

Exterior-releasing Herbs

The term Exterior syndrome indicates, in a broad sense, that the pathogenic change is in the superficial layer of the body. The main characteristic of this change is the conflict between the six exogenous pathogenic factors and the body's resistance, which is represented mainly by the Defensive Qi in the superficial layer of the body. An Exterior syndrome also includes further pathogenic changes of the associated organs, meridians, Qi and Blood.

The Lung is an important organ in Exterior syndrome because it governs the Exterior by dispersing the Defensive Qi to the superficial layer of the body. Moreover, Wind-Heat and Dryness can directly disturb the function of the Lung because they can invade the body through the nose, and not the superficial level.

The main symptoms can be divided into two groups. On the one hand, chills, fever and aversion to cold or wind are present. These are the manifestations in the superficial layer of the body caused by the conflict between pathogenic factors and the Defensive Qi. On the other hand, headache, general pain, thirst, blocked nose, cough and sore throat may be present; these are manifestations caused by disharmony of the circulation of the Qi and Blood in the Bladder meridian and dysfunction of the Lung-Qi.

The purpose of treatment is to expel the exogenous pathogenic factors, and to restore the normal functioning and harmony of all the organs, meridians, Qi and Blood. Methods that can stimulate or strengthen the function of the Defensive Qi or disperse the Lung-Qi and therefore eliminate the pathogenic factors are often used. Other methods, such as promoting Qi and Blood circulation, or regulating the Large Intestine in order to regulate the Lung-Qi, can also be used as assistant procedures in the whole treatment strategy.

Herbs that release the Exterior have the functions of expelling Wind-Cold or Wind-Heat. They are used in conditions where the pathogenic Wind-Cold or Wind-Heat invades the superficial layer of the body.

Pungent or Pungent and Warm

Most of the herbs in this category possess a pungent property. As pungency has a dispersing capacity, the pungent herbs are able to activate Qi movement, open the pores and subcutaneous layer, connect the Exterior with the Interior, disperse the Lung-Qi, harmonize the Nutritive and Defensive systems and therefore expel Wind. Moreover, many of the herbs are pungent and warm in nature. Their functions of activating the Yang and Qi and opening the pores are represented by their induction of sweating in different degrees. Through sweating, Wind and other exogenous pathogenic factors can be eliminated from the superficial layer of the body, therefore stopping the progress of the disease in its primary stage.

Aromatic

Many of the herbs in this category are aromatic, which gives them the ability to open the orifices, penetrate turbidity, spread the pure Qi and transform Dampness. They are therefore used to treat headache, dizziness, nasal obstruction and loss of the sense of smell.

Light in Weight and Gentle in Nature

Many herbs in this category are light in weight and gentle in nature. They mainly enter the Lung and the Bladder meridians, so they are suitable for treating the external pathogenic syndromes that mainly affect those layers and meridians. As wind charac-teristically attacks the upper body, which includes the head, the Lung, the Upper Jiao and the superficial layer of the body, these herbs are often used to treat symptoms such as headache, dizziness, nasal obstruction, runny nose, itchy and painful eyes, cough with or without production, sore throat and general body pain. Many are also used to treat allergies such as hay fever and asthma, as well as many kinds of skin diseases.

What Precautions should be Observed in the usage of Herbs that Release the Exterior?

First of all, since herbs that release the Exterior are pungent and their tendencies of action are ascending and dispersing, especially with the herbs that can cause sweating, overdose may disperse the Qi too much, consume the Yin of the body and cause other complications. In patients who are deficient in Yin or Qi owing to their constitution, chronic disease, stress or dietary habit, these herbs should be used with caution. Fur-thermore, as pungency also has the property of movement, these herbs should also be used with caution in bleeding conditions or in pregnancy.

Secondly, the dosage of herbs should be adjusted to suit the condition of the individ-ual, the syndrome and the season. For elderly people, children, people with a weak constitution and for mild syndromes, in a gentle climate and in the summer, the dosage should be reduced. For adults with a strong constitution and for severe syn-dromes, in a cold winter or a cold place, the dosage should be increased. If sweating must be induced, the dosage is adjusted according to the syndrome. A mild sweat over the whole body is required. Heavy sweating must be avoided because it can only weaken the Qi and Yin.

In the third place, as eliminating Wind-Cold or Wind-Heat is not generally difficult, these herbs should not be used for a long period of time. A dosage of 3 days is rec-ommended to treat Exterior syndrome. If the exogenous pathogenic factors have not been removed completely, then another 3-day dosage can be prescribed. With regard to herbs that may cause heavy sweating, the dosage and treatment course should be adjusted according to the reaction of the patient after each use.

Ma Huang (Ephedrae herba) and Gui Zhi (Cinnamomi cassiae ramulus) can both ex-pel Wind-Cold to treat Exterior Wind-Cold syndrome.

Differences between their Actions and Characteristics

Cautions Regarding their use

Ma Huang and Gui Zhi can expel Wind-Cold and treat Exterior Wind-Cold syndrome. Compared with Gui Zhi, Ma Huang is stronger in inducing sweating and expelling Wind-Cold from the surface of the body. This is because Ma Huang is very pungent and warm, and its speed of movement and strength are stronger than Gui Zhi. When Wind-Cold attacks the body surface, the pores are closed by Cold, which is characteristically contracting, so the Defensive Qi is not able to spread over the surface of the body. In consequence, the patient feels chilly because the surface of the body is not warmed up by the Yang and Qi. The blockage of Defensive Qi inside may then produce Heat and the patient may have a fever. Because Cold initially injures the Yang-Qi in the Greater Yang (Tai Yang) meridian, this stops the Qi circulating freely, and the patient feels pain and stiffness in the back of the body. Due to dysfunction of the dispersion of Lung-Qi, there are also cough and shortness of breath. Ma Huang enters the Lung meridian, disperses the Lung-Qi, enters the Bladder meridian, activates the Defensive Qi, opens the pores, causes sweating and expels Wind and Cold so that the Exterior can be released. This herb is considered as the strongest one for causing sweating. It is the first-line choice where Wind-Cold is severe and the patient has severe chills and fever without sweating, such as in upper respiratory tract infection, cold infections, influenza, acute bronchitis, pneumonia and asthma.

Gui Zhi can also treat Wind-Cold syndrome. Here the therapeutic result is achieved by warming the Blood, promoting Blood circulation, opening up the meridians and activating the Yang-Qi to expel Wind and Cold. Compared with Ma Huang, Gui Zhi is not so warm and pungent, but sweet. It enters the Heart meridian primarily, and the Lung and Bladder meridians secondarily. The warm nature of this herb can reduce Cold in the Blood. Pungency and warmth may also activate the Blood circulation and open up the meridians. The sweetness moderates the warmth and pungency so that the medicinal action may be balanced. As it enters the Lung and Bladder meridians, it can activate the Yang-Qi to eliminate Wind and Cold in the Exterior layer. When the pathogenic Cold is not so severe, the pores are not closed so tightly, which manifests as slight sweating or a milder cold sensation and less pain in the back of the body, Gui Zhi can be used alone. It is especially useful for patients with Exterior syndromes against the background of a Yang-deficient constitution, Bi syndrome or Cold in the Blood, such as in elderly people, patients with chronic bronchitis, pulmonary emphysema, rheumatism or Raynaud's disease.

In clinical practice, Ma Huang and Gui Zhi are often used together to treat severe Wind-Cold syndrome, as they work on different aspects—for instance, the former enters the Qi level, the latter enters the Blood level; the former induces sweating and eliminates Wind-Cold by a short, quick and strong action, the latter promotes the Blood circulation, warms it, stops pain and activates the Yang-Qi in the Blood, thereby expelling Wind-Cold. When they are used together, the therapeutic effects are enhanced.

Although there are differences between Ma Huang and Gui Zhi, they both belong to quite warm and pungent herbs in the herbal group of expelling Wind-Cold. The dosage should be carefully managed. Age, constitution and the present state of health should also be considered. Generally speaking, after taking these herbs, if the patient does not sweat, the dose should be increased within the normal dosage range. If the patient becomes sweaty and the chills and fever are less severe, Ma Huang and Gui Zhi should not be used again. Some herbs with a gentler action can be substituted, such as Jing Jie (Schizonepetae herba) and Fang Feng (Saposhnikoviae radix). If, after a while, the chills and fever return, Ma Huang and Gui Zhi should be used again but in a smaller dosage as the Wind and Cold have already been partially expelled.

Moreover, as the tendency of action of these two herbs is upward and outward, in the following conditions they should not be used or used with caution: patients suffering from acute infection of the nose and throat where there is internal Heat or Heat due to Deficiency in the body, patients suffering from hypertension which indicates a tendency to Liver-Yang rising, or women suffering from menopausal syndrome with hot flushes and night sweats, and people with a Yang constitution or with heart disease, because these herbs can increase the contraction of the cardiac muscle and increase oxygen consumption, which makes the heart overwork.

Differences between the Actions of Ma Huang, Zhi Ma Huang and Ma Huang Gen

Ma Huang is also called Sheng Ma Huang. 'S heng' means 'raw'. Sheng Ma Huang is very pungent and warm. It is a very strong herb used to expel Wind and Cold to release Exterior Wind-Cold syndrome. As Sheng Ma Huang is pungent and hot, the dosage should be controlled and it should not be used over a long period of time. Overdose may cause heavy sweating, which injures the Yin, Body Fluids and Qi. It should be used with caution, especially in patients with a weak constitution and Deficiency syndrome. As its actions have an upward and outward tendency, Ma Huang should not be used or used with caution in cases of hypertension and heart disease.

Zhi Ma Huang is gentler in action compared with Sheng Ma Huang, because roasting with honey moderates the pungent taste. Zhi Ma Huang acquires the nature of honey, which is sweet and moistening, so its dispersing action is not as strong and quick as that of Sheng Ma Huang. It is often used to disperse the Lung-Qi and cause it to descend, to moisten the Lung and stop wheezing. In clinical practice, it is often used for treating asthma, bronchitis, pneumonia and acute nephritis.

Ma Huang Gen has completely different characteristics from both Sheng Ma Huang and Zhi Ma Huang. It is neutral, sweet and astringent, and enters the Lung meridian. It is excellent for stopping sweating. It can be used for treating spontaneous sweating and night sweating. It treats only the symptoms however, so it is often combined with other herbs that treat the cause of sweating. In addition, it should not be used in the syndrome of Phlegm accumulation or Exterior syndrome because it has an astringent property, which can retain Phlegm, close the pores and retain the pathogenic factors within the body.

Characteristic Functions of Gui Zhi

'Twig of plants enters the limbs of human body': Such similes and allegories were often used in ancient times in Chinese medicine to explain the complicated links between the human and the natural environment. Gui Zhi is an example of this. This herb is the twig of the plant and has a warm, pungent and sweet nature. Besides expelling Wind and Cold to treat Exterior syndrome, Gui Zhi is often used to treat Bi syndrome. In this case, it can relieve pain and cold sensations in the affected limbs or joints. The therapeutic effects are achieved by warming and strengthening the Heart-Yang, promoting the Blood circulation, spreading the Yang-Qi and unblocking the meridians, especially in the limbs. This is why it is often used in Bi syndrome caused by blockage of the circulation of Qi and Blood by Wind, Dampness or Cold; examples are rheumatic fever, rheumatoid arthritis, rheumatic heart disease, Raynaud's disease and the early and mid-phases of vasculitis.

In chronic diseases, when internal Cold blocks the meridians, a small amount (about 10 m) of Gui Zhi alcohol drink is also a preferred formulation for daily use in the diet. Soaking 15 grams of Gui Zhi in a liter of alcohol (about 40% alcohol) made from cereals for 6 weeks yields Gui Zhi alcohol drink. Alcohol is pungent and warm, so is considered to have the functions of invigorating the Blood and unblocking the meridians. The functions of Gui Zhi and alcohol therefore enhance each other. It is commonly used for chronic Bi syndrome.

As Gui Zhi is pungent and warm, it should be used with caution if there is any deficiency of Yin with Empty-Fire or Liver-Yang rising in the syndrome or in the treatment of Heat-type Bi syndrome.

Jing Jie (Schizonepetae herba) and Fang Feng (Saposhnikoviae radix) are often used for Exterior Wind-Cold syndrome.

Differences between using Ma Huang and Gui Zhi

Jing Jie and Fang Feng are both pungent and warm. However, they are far gentler than Ma Huang and Gui Zhi. They can expel Wind and Cold and are commonly used for mild Exterior Wind-Cold syndrome. In regions with temperate climates, where Wind and Cold do not close the pores tightly, they are more often applied than Ma Huang and Gui Zhi for cold infections, influenza, certain stages of infectious childhood diseases and some skin diseases in which Exterior syndromes are involved. Meanwhile, they are also often used with pungent-cold herbs in syndromes where Wind-Heat is mixed with Wind-Cold. The patient may have symptoms such as chills, fever, thirst, sore throat and general pain. These two herbs are more often used in combination with cold herbs than Ma Huang and Gui Zhi.

Comparing Jing Jie with Fang Feng, Jing Jie is lighter and more dispersing. It is pungent but not strong, slightly warm but not dry. It is especially good at expelling Wind, no matter whether it is Wind-Cold or Wind-Heat. Moreover, it can expel Wind from the Blood so is often used in skin disorders when there is itching caused by Wind invasion, for instance in eczema, urticaria and food allergy. It is also used for infectious childhood diseases with Exterior syndrome and skin eruptions, such as measles, rubella, scarlet fever, chickenpox and so on.

Fang Feng is sweet, pungent and warm and enters the Bladder, Lung and Spleen meridians. As its sweet taste moderates the pungent taste, it is less strong in dispersing Wind on the surface of the body than Jing Jie. However, as it is warmer than Jing Jie and enters the Spleen meridian, it is especially good at expelling Dampness and Cold in the layers below the body surface, such as the subcutaneous region and muscles, which are controlled by the Spleen. When the patient feels pain and heaviness of the muscles, Fang Feng is more suitable than Jing Jie. This is also the reason that Fang Feng is more often used in Bi syndromes.

Although both herbs are gentle, they do have a pungent and warm nature, so both should be used with caution in patients without Wind invasion or in Yin deficiency with Empty-Heat.

Differences between the Actions of Jing Jie, Jing Jie Sui, Chao Jin Jie and Jing Jie Tan

Generally speaking, Jing Jie Sui is more thin-pungent than Jing Jie as it is the bud, which is believed to be lighter in nature. It has a quicker and lighter action in expelling Wind. It is used at the very beginning of Wind-Cold syndrome or Wind-Heat syndrome.

Comparing raw with roasted Jing Jie, raw Jing Jie is more pungent. It is used for Exterior Wind-Cold syndrome when sweating is not present, which means that the pores are closed. It can open the pores, cause mild sweating and expel Wind and Cold. Roasted Jing Jie is less pungent because processing has reduced the taste. If the pores are open, sweating is present, or the patient has an aversion to wind instead of cold; this indicates that it is not necessary to open the pores, so roasted Jing Jie is then more suitable.

Jing Jie Tan is able to stop bleeding and it is used in bleeding conditions. When Jing Jie is roasted to charcoal, its pungent property is reduced, but an astringent property emerges. It can stabilize the Blood and stop bleeding. Meanwhile, it can also expel Wind and calm the Blood, therefore stopping bleeding.

Xiang Ru/Summer Ma Huang

'Xiang' means 'aroma', 'fragrance'; ' Ru' means 'gentle'. As the name explains, this herb is pungent and slightly warm with an aromatic smell. It enters the Spleen, Stomach and Lung meridians. Xiang Ru can, on the one hand, disperse Wind and Cold, induce sweating and release the Exterior; on the other hand, it transforms Dampness and harmonizes the Spleen and Stomach. The functions are similar to that of Ma Huang, but gentler. It is often used in summer when the weather is warm, the Wind-Cold is not so strong, the pores are not closed so tightly as in winter and the mild Wind-Cold attacks the body and causes an Exterior Wind-Cold syndrome. Meanwhile, Xiang Ru is used to treat abdominal pain, vomiting and diarrhea in summer, if overconsumption of cold drinks has injured the Stomach and Spleen, such as in acute gastritis.

Heat-clearing Chinese Herbs

TCM theory states that the occurrence of the disease depends on the interaction between zheng qi (nonpathogenic qi) and xie qi (pathogenic qi). The idea of disease is the struggle between pathogenic qi and nonpathogenic qi; in this struggle process, there will be changes between yin and yang. TCM holds that variation between the evil aspect and healthy trend determines the occurrence of disease. Therefore, in TCM, inflammatory and antimicrobial therapy lies in strengthening the healthy trend and dispelling the evil aspect in order to keep a balanced state between yin and yang.

Herbal medicine is one of the main components of TCM which has long been used for its multiple types of disease treatment. In recent times, it is making a rapid progress in scientific investigation and attracting great attention due to the good therapeutic effects and minimal side effects of the herbs. Chinese herbs used in the treatment of diseases are grouped into many categories. One of these is heat-clearing Chinese herbs (HCCHs). Herbs in this group are mostly cold in nature and can clear away heat, purge fire, dry dampness, cool blood, and relieve toxic material. Their main action is clearing away interior heat, and thus they are considered to be antipyretic. Because of all these properties, HCCHs may be effective in the treatment of inflammatory disease and microbial infection.

Scutellaria Baicalensis

Scutellaria baicalensis is a species of flowering plant belonging to Lamiaceae family It is a heat-clearing, phlegm-removing herb, traditionally used to cool heat, drain fire, clear damp-heat, stop bleeding, calm the fetus, and descend yang. The dry root part of Sc. baicalensis has many pharmacological effects including antipyretic, hepatoprotective, antihypertensive, diuretic, and antibiotic activities. It is mildly sedating and also used to treat dysentery and chronic hepatitis. Sc. baicalensis has distinct effects in the treatment of inflammatory diseases; it alleviates inflammation by decreasing the expression of interleukin (IL)-1b, IL-6, and IL-12, and the production of tumor necrosis factor (TNF)-α and soluble intercellular adhesion molecule-1 (ICAM-1). In Xie xin herbal decoction, huang qin, in combination with huang lian, inhibits nitric oxide (NO) production in vitro and in vivo in lipopolysaccharide (LPS)-stimulated RAW264.7 cells. Oroxylin A, which is a flavonoid found in dried root of Sc. baicalensis, has also shown good anti-inflammatory effect. Moreover, Sc. baicalensis has antibacterial effect against Helicobacter pylori as well as inhibits the growth of Escherichia coli B, coagulase-negative staphylococci, and Saccharomyces cerevisiae.

Coptis Chinensis

Coptis chinensis belongs to Ranunculaceae family. Traditionally, it has been used to drain fire, detoxify and disinfect, stop bleeding, cure eczema, burns, and ulcer, and to descend yang. The main pharmacodynamic properties have long been recognized in the treatment of intestinal infections including acute gastroenteritis, cholera, and bacillary dysentery. It also used for treating various diseases including skin diseases, conjunctivitis, otitis, and hypertension. C. chinensis has been demonstrated to have anti-inflammatory effects through different mechanisms. It inhibits TNF-induced Nuclear factor-kappaB (NF-kB) signaling in human keratinocytes by blocking the NF-kB–dependent pathway. It also decreases Th17 cytokine secretion and differentiation by activation of extracellular signal-regulated protein kinases 1 and 2 (ERK1/2) and down-regulation of phosphorylated signal transducer and activator of transcription 3 (p-STAT3) and retinoic acid-related orphan receptor γt (RORγt) expression. It also reduces Th1 cytokine secretion and differentiation by inhibition of protein 38 (p38) mitogen activated protein kinase (MAPK) and Jun N-terminal kinase (JNK) activation along with down-regulation of STAT1 and STAT4 activities.

In combination with other herbs, C. chinensis exhibited a good anti-inflammatory effect; the ethanol extract from Zuojin Pill inhibited inducible nitric oxide synthase (iNOS), cyclooxygenase 2 (COX-2), IL-6, IL-1β, and TNF-α expression by preventing the nuclear translocation of the NF-κB p50 and p65 subunits in RAW 264.7 cells. Another Chinese medicinal formula, IBS-20, containing C. chinensis decreased LPS-stimulated pro-inflammatory cytokine secretion from JAWS II dendritic cells and also blocked the interferon gamma (IFNγ)-induced drop in transepithelial electric resistance which is an index of permeability, in fully differentiated Caco-2 monolayer. C. chinensis has also significant antimicrobial activity against a variety of microorganisms including bacteria, viruses, fungi, protozoans, helminths, and Chlamydia, including Staphylococcus aureus, Pseudomonas aeruginosa, E. coli, Propionibacterium acnes, Streptococcus pneumoniae, Vibrio cholerae, Bacillus anthracis, Bacillus dysenteriae, and Sa. cerevisiae. Berberine, the major active component of C. chinensis, was found to be bactericidal on V. cholera and capable of inhibiting bacterial adherence to mucosal or epithelial surfaces.

Flos Lonicerae

Flos lonicerae is a honeysuckle flower belonging to Caprifoliaceae family. It is a widely used herb in China for the treatment of infection by exopathogenic wind-heat or epidemic febrile diseases. The dried flower and buds of Flos Lonicerae have shown various pharmacological effects including anti-nociceptive, anti-diabetic, anti-tumor, antioxidant, anti-angiogenic, antipyretic, antiviral, and hepatoprotective activities. Flos Lonicerae demonstrated anti-inflammatory properties through suppression of mediator release from the mast cells activated by secretagogues. In addition, the n-butanol fraction containing Flos Lonicerae can alleviate inflammation better than celecoxib in carrageen- and croton oil-induced paw edema and ear edema. Flos Lonicerae contains various active compounds that have marked anti-inflammatory effect, including luteolin (suppresses inflammatory mediator release by blocking NF-kB and MAPKs pathway activation in HMC-11 cells), chlorogenic acid (inhibits rat reflux esophagitis induced by pylorus and forestomach ligation), and loncerin (reduces edema by suppressing T cell proliferation, NO production from the macrophages, and shifting cellular immunity from Th1- toward Th2-type responses). Flos Lonicerae has significant antimicrobial activity against diverse species of bacteria and fungi. It has inhibitory effect against H. pylori and Porphyromonas gingivalis, and it treats candidal septic arthritis. It also has antimicrobial effect against oral pathogens including Streptococcus mutans, Actinomyces viscosus, and Bacteroides melaninogenicus.

Forsythia Suspensa

Forsythia suspensa is a flowering plant belonging to the family Oleaceae. Traditionally, it used to treat carbuncle, disperse lumps, and stagnation, and to expel wind and heat. The fruit of F. suspensa has potent pharmacological actions such as antiviral, choleretic, antipyretic, hepatoprotective, antiemetic, and diuretic effects. F. suspensa alleviates inflammation by reducing the anaphylactic antibodies, mast cell degranulation, and histamine release. It also significantly suppresses β-conglycinin–induced T lymphocyte proliferation and IL-4 synthesis. F. suspensa fruit inhibits NO production and iNOS gene expression by its active components rengyolone, dibenzylbutyrolactone lignans, as well as its butanol fraction of the aqueous extract. It also inhibits TNF-α and COX-2 production. Another bioactive agent, arctigenin, inhibits increase in capillary permeability and leukocyte recruitment into inflamed tissues, by reduction of the vascular leakage and cellular events through inhibition of production of inflammatory mediators such as NO and pro-inflammatory cytokines such as IL-1b, IL-6, TNF-α, and prostaglandin E_2 (PGE2). Moreover, F. suspensa inhibits NF-kB nucleus translocation through reduction in I-kappa-B (IkB) phosphorylation and suppression of NF-kB–regulated proteins, and also reduces the activation of MAPKs. Various studies have reported the antimicrobial effect of F. suspensa. It has potent antibacterial activity against E. coli, Sta. aureus, Bacillus subtilis, Str. mutans, and Po. gingivalis and antifungal activity against Aspergillus flavus, Rhizopus stolonifer, Penicillium citrinum, Aspergillus niger, and Saccharomyces carlsbergensis. F. suspensa suppresses influenza A virus–induced RANTES secretion by human bronchial epithelial cells to stop accumulation of inflammatory cells in the infective sites, which has been reported to play a crucial role in the progression of chronic inflammation and multiple sclerosis after viral infection.

Isatidis Folium

Isatidis folium is a flowering plant belonging to the family Brassicaceae. The leaves of Isatidis Folium are traditionally used for the treatment of sore throat, redness of skin, and as an antipyretic. Isatidis Folium has also been used to treat encephalitis, acute dysentery, hepatitis, measles, pneumonia, influenza, epidemic cerebrospinal meningitis, encephalitis B, viral pneumonia, mumps, and diabetics. Tryptanthrin, an alkaloid isolated from Isatidis leaves, has shown anti-inflammatory effect due to its strong inhibitory effect on the COX-2 enzyme. Several derivatives of hydroxycinnamic acid, including ferulic acid and sinapic acid, are also thought to be important to inhibit inflammation.Isatidis Folium possesses valuable viricidal effect in the control of pseudorabies infection in swine.

Radix Isatidis

Isatidis radix belongs to the family Brassicaceae. Traditionally, it used to cool blood. The dry root of Isatidis Radix has many pharmacological activities such as antibiotic, anti-diabetic, and immune-stimulating effects and is used to treat encephalitis B and viral infections. Methanolic extracts of Isatidis Radix can significantly inhibit the release of inflammatory mediators from the macrophages, such as NO, PGE2, and pro-inflammatory cytokines. Isatidis Radix has also been demonstrated to suppress the growth of E. coli and H. pylori and increases blood neutrophil phagocytosis of ^{32}P-labeled Sta. aureus. Syringic acid isolated from Isatidis Radix inhibited LPS-induced endotoxin shock. Besides, Isatidis Radix is found to be clinically effective against the infections caused by various subtypes and strains of influenza viruses including Severe Acute Respiratory Syndrome (SARS).

Viola Yedoensis

Viola yedoensis is a flowering plant belonging to the violet family of Violaceae. Traditionally, it used to cool heat, and disinfect and detoxify. V. yedoensis has several pharmacological effects including antibiotic, anti-inflammatory, and antipyretic activities. It can also be used for the treatment of skin diseases, i.e. eczema, impetigo, acne, pruritus, and cradle cap, and for upper respiratory tract infections with fever. It has been reported to have antimicrobial activity against B. subtilis, Str. mutans, and Po. gingivalis. It inhibits the replication of herpes simplex virus-1 and enterovirus 71 in the human neuroblastoma SK-N-SH cell line. Cyclotides from Viola are shown to be effective in inhibiting human immunodeficiency virus (HIV) replication.

Pulsatilla Radix

Pulsatilla radix is a medicinal root plant of the Ranunculaceae. It used to cool heat, disinfect and detoxify, and clear damp-heat in TCM. The root of Pulsatilla Radix has anti-inflammatory, antiparasitic, and antimicrobial action. It can treat dyspepsia, premenstrual tension, and psychosomatic disturbances. A quinine-type compound, pulsaquinone, isolated from the aqueous ethanol extract of the roots of Pulsatilla Radix exhibited antimicrobial activities against an anaerobic non–spore-forming gram-positive bacillus, Pr. acnes, which is related to the pathogenesis of the inflamed lesions in a common skin disease, acne vulgaris. Moreover, 4-hydroxy-3-methoxycinnamic acid of Pulsatilla Radix is found to have a selective growth inhibitor of the human intestinal bacteria, Clostridium perfringens and E. coli.

Andrographis Paniculata

Andrographis paniculata is also known as nemone chinensi and belongs to Acanthaceae family. The active compounds isolated from An. paniculata, including diterpene, lactone, and andrographolide, have shown anti-inflammatory, anti-allergic, immune-stimulatory, and antiviral activities.An. paniculata alleviates inflammation by inhibiting iNOS, TNF-α, IL-1b, IL-6, and IL-12 expression and NO production by down-regulation of p38MAPKs signaling pathways. It also suppresses influenza A virus-induced RANTES secretion by human bronchial epithelial cells.

Houttuynia Cordata

Houttuynia cordata is one of the two species in the genus Houttuynia and belongs to the family Saururaceae. It has many pharmacological effects including immune-stimulating, anti-inflammatory, antibiotic, antiviral, diuretic, analgesic, and hemostatic effects. It also used to treat pneumonia, bronchitis, colitis, urogenital tract infections, and chronic obstructive respiratory diseases, and topically to treat herpes simplex.

Patrinia Herba

Patrinia herba is a medicinal herb belongs to family of Valerianaceae. It has antibiotic, hepatoprotective, sedating, and hypnotic effects, and it can be used to treat mumps. Patrinia Herba can inhibit adjuvant-induced inflammation and hyperalgesia. In rats, it attenuates Freund's adjuvant (CFA)–induced hyperalgesia and facilitates the recovery from hyperalgesia, and also reduces edema.

Warming Herbs

"Interior cold" is a condition either caused by invasion of external cold pathogen or an internally developed condition. In both cases - as the name of the pathology suggests the condition, the experience, the symptoms of "internal cold" is the feeling of cold.

External invasion of cold pathogen develops by residing long term in a cold environment and chronically exposing the body to cold atmosphere and surfaces. Internally developed "cold" is the result of organ deficiencies, specifically deficiency of Qi (energy) and Yang (the body's warming faculty). Every body organ owns Qi and Yang (as well as Yin and Blood). Deficiency of Qi will lead to lack of energy and tiredness, but if the condition worsens and the Yang becomes deficient "cold" symptoms develop. Usually the organs that predominantly suffer from Yang deficiency are the Spleen (in traditional Chinese medicine the Spleen is referred to as the collective work of some organs and systems participating in the digestion rather than the anatomical organ spleen), and the Kidney. In the case of Spleen Yang deficiency there is coldness in the abdomen, while in Kidney Yang deficiency there is coldness in the back. Spleen Yang deficiency furthermore manifests with symptoms of deficient digestion such as watery stools that contain undigested food. Kidney Yang deficiency manifests in loose stools, frequent urination, poor sexual desire, sterility (in TCM the Kidney governs both the urinary and the reproductive systems). In both pathologies there are cold hands and feet, overall feeling of cold, fear of cold.

Major Chinese Herbs

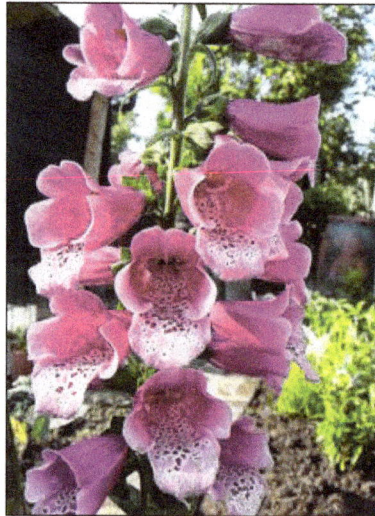

A very famous Chinese herb that strongly warms the interior and enters the Spleen and Kidney channels is Fu Zi (Aconitum carmicaeli). It restores devastated Yang where the warming faculty is extremely weak. As it enters the Spleen and Kidney it benefits Spleen/Kidney Yang deficiency disorders. Additionally it enters the Heart, boosts the circulation and strengthens the vessels. It is also a very good herb for joint pain/swelling/numbness, especially the kind that gets worse when exposed to cold.

Another major herb that warms the interior is Wu Zhu Yu (Evodia rutaecarpa). It is one of the herbs that has the ability to lead the energy downward, being very beneficial for rebellious Qi symptoms such as vomiting and acid reflux, as well as sores of the mouth and tongue.

There is an interesting story about how the herb was named. Back in Ancient China there used to be a custom that the smaller kingdom had to pay tribute to the larger kingdom in order to keep the peace. One time the small Wu kingdom brought the larger and stronger Chu kingdom their national herb, called "Herb of Wu kingdom", as a present. A doctor with the name Dr. Zhu planted the herb. After the king of the Chu kingdom suffered sever abdominal pain and was successfully cured with this herb, he embraced the herb and changed it's name from "Herb of Wu kingdom" to "Wu-Zhu's fruit". "Wu" - because it came from the Wu kingdom, "Zhu" because it was planted in his kingdom by Dr. Zhu, and "fruit" because it was a fruit. Ever since the herb is referred to by this name – Wu Zhu Yu.

Fresh ginger is warm herb that benefits the first stages of common cold. When dried it's temperature changes from warm to hot and the herb is now used in the "warm interior" class herbs. Gan Jiang (Zingiber officinale) rescues devastated Yang, warms the Lungs and transforms "cold phlegm". It also stops bleeding due to cold.

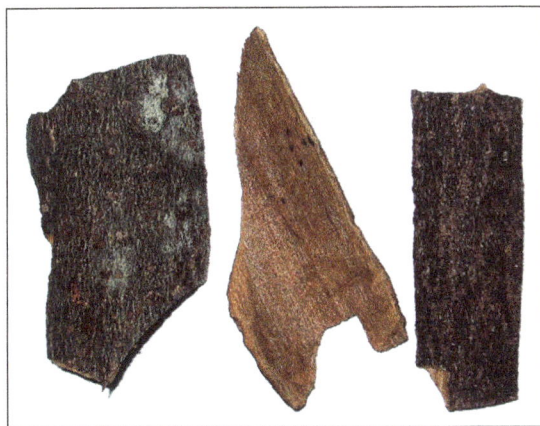

Rou Gui (Cinnamomum cassia) – cinnamon bark – strongly reinforces the Yang and brings it back to its source. It also warms the channels, unblocks the channels and vessels and promotes the movement of energy throughout the body. Simultaneously it aids the generation of energy and blood in the body and is often used together with herbs that tonify the Qi and blood.

Another herb that warms the channels and alleviates pain is Dou Chi Jiang (Litsea cubeba). It is particularly good for painful menstruation due to cold. Xiao Hui Xiang (Foeniculum vulgare) – warms and encourages movement in the Liver channel, benefiting hernia disorders, as they manifest from "cold in the Liver channel". Ding Xiang (Eugenia caryophyllata) – warms the Kidneys and benefits the Yang, thus is used for impotence or clear vaginal discharge, caused by Kidney Yang deficiency. Chuan Jiao (Zanthoxylum bungeanum) besides warming the interior kills parasites, and is used for roundworms. Bi Ba (Piper longum) can be topically applied for toothache.

Qi-regulating Herbs

In traditional Chinese medicine the Liver is the organ that governs the smooth flow of Qi throughout the whole person. To be in a good state of health – physically and emotionally - one needs to have a smooth, uninterrupted flow of energy in both body and mind. When the Qi flows continuously and in the proper direction the body organs function properly and the overall physical and psychological states are harmonious. If the Qi ceases to flow smoothly one becomes unbalanced on both mental and physical levels. Since the Liver governs the smooth flow of Qi when the Qi stagnates the Liver becomes unbalanced. And vice versa - if the Liver is unbalanced - the Qi, which is controlled by the Liver, will stagnate. In both cases this diagnosis is called "Liver Qi stagnation". Symptoms of Liver Qi stagnation are distention or pain under the ribs and tender breasts in women, caused by the energy blockage. On emotional level Liver Qi stagnation manifests in depression, irritability and mood changes.

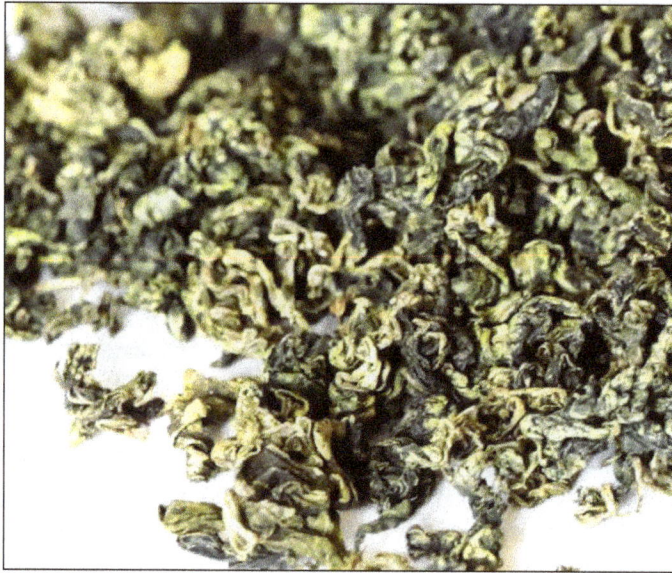

When the Liver becomes stagnated and overactive he turns into a bad neighbor and starts assaulting other organs and systems. His biggest victim is the Spleen - the collective work of some organs and systems, participating in the digestion not really the anatomical organ spleen. When the Liver "overacts" the Spleen symptoms include poor appetite, abdominal distention, epigastric pain, feeling of pulsation in the epigastrium, sour regurgitation, nausea, belching, diarrhea or constipation. Another victim of the Liver is the Lung. When the Liver assaults the Lung the Qi of the Lung stagnates manifesting in symptoms such as stifling sensation in the chest, sensation that inhaling is insufficient, coughing, wheezing, labored breathing.

The herbs used in this category have moving quality and address one or more of the organs affected by Qi stagnation. They are rarely used alone and are often combined with herbs that address other pathologies which usually accompany Qi stagnation.

Major Chinese Herbs

Two main herbs used to move the Qi in Chinese medicine are peels of tangerine. Chen

Pi and Qing Pi (both belonging to Citrus reticulata) are aged peel and green peel of tangerine. Chen Pi benefits the Spleen/Stomach partnership and the Lung, and relieves Qi stagnation symptoms in these organs. It also dries dampness and is very useful for phlegm in the Lung (productive cough) and dampness in the Spleen (poor energy, feeling of heaviness, fatigue, loose stool). Qing Pi on the other hand enters the Liver/Gall Bladder partnership and benefits Qi stagnation in the Liver, manifesting in symptoms such as distention and pain under the ribs, or hernial pain. As it also dries dampness it is used for damp-phlegm with malarial disorders.

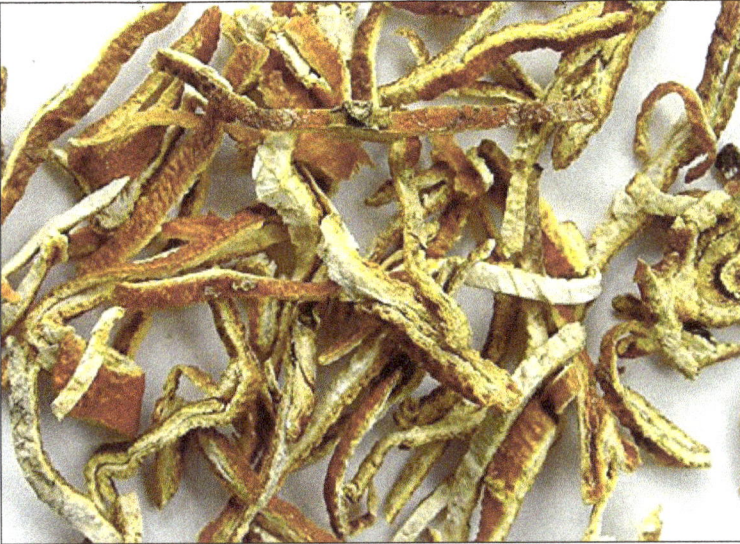

Another herb that is derived from citrus fruit is Zhi Shi (Citrus aurantium). The immature fruit of bitter orange moves Qi and also directs the Qi downwards, making it very beneficial for constipation due to Qi stagnation. Being a citrus herb it also benefits phlegm and is used to clear phlegm from the chest and epigastrium. Fo Shou (Citrus medica) is a fourth citrus herb in this category. The finger citron fruit harmonizes the Qi in all organs that suffer from Qi stagnation – the Liver, the Lung, the Stomach and the Spleen. Just like the other citrus herbs it also dries dampness and transforms phlegm.

Four herbs in this class contain the character "xiang". "Xiang" means "incense" if we translate it as a noun or "fragrant/aromatic" if we translate it as an adjective. Xiang Fu (Cyperus rotundus) - "aromatic appendage" is an intensely moving herb, used for Liver Qi stagnation, especially in gynecological disorders caused by this pathology, such as painful or irregular menstruation. Mu Xiang (Aucklandia lappa) translates to "wood fragrance" and benefits as well as prevents Qi stagnation, therefore is used together with tonifying herbs, as they can be heavy and stagnating. Chen Xiang (Aquilaria agallocha) - "sinking fragrance" and Tan Xiang (Santalum album) – heartwood of sandalwood are aromatic herbs that both promote the movement of energy and ease pain.

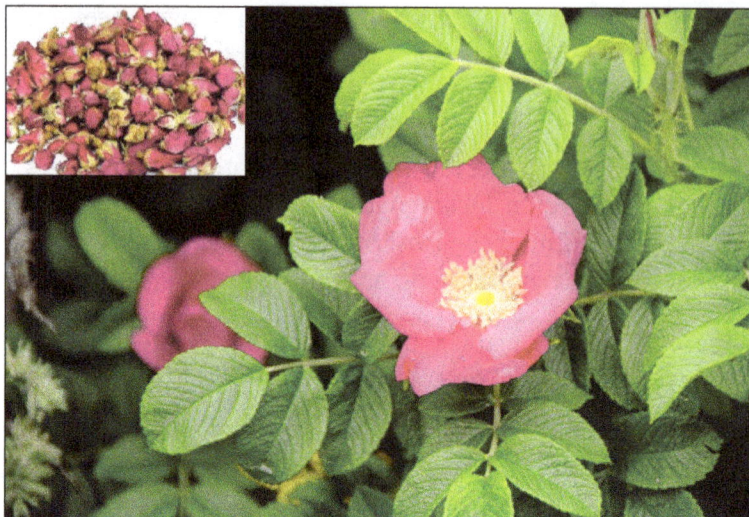

Mei Gui Hua (Rosa Rugosa) - Chinese rose - is picked when the flowers have just opened. It moves Qi and also moves blood, thus is good for menstrual pain due to blood stasis or blood stasis caused by trauma. Chuan Lian Zi (Melia toosendan) is pagoda tree fruit that moves Qi but being toxic it also kills roundworms and tapeworms. Li Zhi He (Litchi chinesis) – the delicious Lychee nut, native to southern China, Taiwan, Bangladesh and Southeast Asia but now known throughout the whole world, regulates the Qi in the Liver and Stomach and is beneficial for testicular and hernia pain. Xie Bai (Allium macrostemon) – macrostem onion – is a warming herb that warms the chest and expels turbid phlegm, Da Fu Pi (Areca catechu) – areca peel – dries dampness, especially in the Stomach and Intestines.

Phlegm-resolving Herbs

Phlegm is a product of the body's activities acting upon qi and moisture taken in with food and beverages; it is "congealed moisture." Unlike qi, phlegm is always viewed by Chinese physicians as substantive and stagnating rather than light and flowing, though there are two kinds of phlegm: the visible, which has greater accumulation of matter, and the invisible, which is finely divided, though not as fine as qi. Phlegm is, in some ways, comparable to another body humor, blood, which is also produced by the body's activities acting upon qi, and is a sticky substance that shares some of the same potential pathologies with phlegm: deficiency, inadequate circulation, firm coagulation, and complexing with heat or cold factors.

Phlegm is a normal and required substance in terms of the mucous membrane lining and other lubricating functions, but it becomes a pathological substance when:

•   It is derived from stagnated food in the stomach;

- When normal phlegm (mucoid substance) is produced in excess; or

- When it is complexed with internal or external pathological factors, such as cold, heat, wind, or toxin.

Phlegm accumulates when the lungs are irritated, when the moisture of the body is overheated by pathological qi (causing it to dry and transform into thick phlegm), when the qi is stagnant and the normal phlegm is not circulated (or when pathological phlegm is not eliminated quickly due to poor circulation of the fluid), and when the kidneys are too cold and the moisture condenses and transforms into phlegm. Phlegm may become insufficient when there is an inadequate source of the necessary nutrients in the diet; when the spleen is weak and cannot raise the qi derived from food upward to moisturize the upper body; when the lungs suffer from deficient qi and cannot transform moisture to phlegm; or when the environmental conditions or the consumption of drying foods (such as spices) disperse too much of the existing phlegm.

Phlegm is thought to have a similarity to grease or fat, and therefore, fatty foods are deemed one potential source of phlegm. In general, any food that is not completely digested is said to give rise only to a pathological type of phlegm: normal phlegm is produced when pure substances are obtained from digested foods and then processed into a useful body lubricant. Obese persons are said to be displaying an excess of phlegm in their extra body weight: The equivalence of phlegm, fatty foods, and body fat is most clearly demonstrated by this connection. According to Chinese thinking, the spleen and lungs have the primary responsibility for generating and circulating the mucoid substances necessary for normal body functions, and dysfunctions of these organs are often responsible for the accumulation of fats.

While most Westerners think of phlegm as referring only to the excess mucus produced in the lungs and sinuses, from the Oriental view, phlegm can exist in many places in the body; it may form lumps, it may block the meridians, obstruct the heart orifices, or simply accumulate throughout the tissues, preventing the normal in and out flow of qi.

Soft or fluid-filled swellings in the body are generally regarded as phlegm masses. This would include lymphatic swellings, ovarian cysts, thyroid nodules, lipomas, and breast lumps that are not hardened; some of these are malignant masses. The thickened fluid obstructing the bursa of the joints in patients with bursitis is considered a phlegm disorder. Symptoms of phlegm accumulation associated with the digestive system include nausea, vomiting, and greasy stool.

Phlegm and retained fluids are pathological products of impaired local or general water metabolism. The concept of phlegm (tan) and phlegm-fluid retention (tanyin) in Chinese medicine embraces a wide range of manifestations. Phlegm and phlegm fluids are either substantial or non-substantial. Substantial phlegm and retained fluids are visible. Non-substantial phlegm and retained fluids refer to pathological manifestations such as dizziness, nausea, vomiting, shortness of breath, palpitations, or mania and semi-consciousness, all of which are linked to invisible phlegm or fluid discharge from the body. Nonetheless, these conditions respond well when treated as substantial phlegm and retained fluids. Phlegm and retained fluids are caused by the influence of the six exogenous pathogenic factors, irregular diet, or abnormal emotional activities; all impair the water metabolism of the lung, spleen, kidney, and triple burner qi. The lung dominates the dispersion and descent of qi and the distribution of body fluids. The water retention resulting from a failure of these functions produces phlegm and retained fluids. The spleen controls the transportation and transformation of water, the failure of which causes an accumulation of water which then turns into phlegm and other retained fluids. The kidney is responsible for the gassification of water [steaming the water; converting water to qi]. When kidney yang is insufficient, water cannot be transformed into qi. It accumulates and, again, turns into phlegm and other retained fluids. Retained fluids and phlegm may also appear when the triple burner passages are blocked, for the normal transportation, distribution, and excretion of body fluids are interfered with. Furthermore, since the triple burner houses all the zangfu organs, failure of the qi activity of the triple burner may result in the formation of pathogenic phlegm and retained fluids and make them accumulate in the zangfu organs and, more superficially, in the tendons, bones, skin, and muscles, causing various pathological changes.

The diagnosis of phlegm or fluid retention syndrome often revolves around three factors: a moist, and, especially, a thick tongue coating; a smooth, and, especially, a full, slippery pulse; and obvious signs of phlegm accumulation, such as discharge of excess sputum (lung/sinus problems), obesity, palpable soft accumulations (lumps and swellings), and adverse reactions to intake of greasy foods. However, because phlegm retention can occur in persons with a wide range of accompanying conditions, and because phlegm retention can be of the "non-substantial" type, one may need to look further. Some examples of manifestation of phlegm disorder are mentioned in the as follows:

> "Phlegm that blocks the lungs results in coughing, asthmatic breathing, and expectoration of sputum. Phlegm in the heart causes suffocating feeling in the chest and palpitations. If the Heart Meridian [heart orifices] is obstructed by phlegm, dementia and loss of consciousness may occur. If the heart is disturbed by phlegm-fire, mania may occur. Phlegm stagnating in the stomach causes nausea, vomiting, and fullness in the stomach. An accumulation of phlegm in the meridians, tendons, and bones may cause scrofula, subcutaneous nodules, a numbness of the limbs, hemiplegia, or fistulous infection of the tissues. Phlegm attacking the head produces dizziness. Phlegm and qi in the throat may produce the sensation of a foreign body in the throat. Retention of fluids also has different syndromes. Morbid fluid in the intestine produces a gurgling sound. In the costal region, it produces a full sensation in the chest and pain on coughing. If it accumulates in the diaphragm, it causes stuffiness in the chest, coughing,

dyspnea, difficulty in lying flat, and puffiness. Morbid fluid in the tissues and skin causes edema, absence of sweat, and heavy feeling of the body."

Herbs that help resolve phlegm problems are divided, in the Materia Medica, into those which resolve cold phlegm (which is moist, thin, and clear), and those which resolve hot phlegm (which is drier, thick, and sometimes discolored). In most cases, herbs from both categories are combined together in varying proportions to get the best influences of the important phlegm-resolving herbs; several herbs from other Materia Medica categories have phlegm-resolving properties, and may be included in developing an optimal prescription. In the following presentation, the two main groups (herbs for resolving hot phlegm and herbs for resolving cold-phlegm) are listed in accordance with Oriental Materia Medica (Hsu) with some adjustments from Thousand Formulas and Thousand Herbs of Traditional Chinese Medicine (Huang and Wang).

Along with the description of each herb, an example of a formula in which it is utilized is offered to help illustrate the principles of combining that have been relied upon in China. It will be noted that many of the formulas contain citrus materials: citrus (chenpi), aurantium (jupi), chih-shih (zhishi), or blue citrus (qingpi). These herbs are found in the qi-regulating section of the Materia Medica, but they are important herbs for resolving phlegm accumulations, both because of inherent phlegm-resolving activity of the herbs and because of the principle: "if the qi circulates well, phlegm also circulates." Ginger (fresh ginger, shengjiang) also appears in many of the formulas because it helps to resolve phlegm and to promote the stomach function so that food stagnation does not arise. In addition, several of the formulas contain herbs for clearing heat (e.g., scute, gardenia, anemarrhena); their use is indicated in cases where heat pathogens combine with or cause phlegm accumulation and it also is important when prolonged phlegm accumulation turns to heat. Several of the formulas contain herbs for dispelling wind (notably siler, angelica, chiang-huo, asarum, and schizonepeta) to help treat acute ailments or the surface manifestation of a chronic ailment, and some formulas contain tonic herbs (e.g., ginseng, jujube, licorice, atractylodes, and hoelen) to aid the spleen in transforming and transporting functions so that phlegm does not continue to accumulate. When the phlegm is in the lungs, herbs that reduce coughing may also be included (e.g., apricot seed, perilla seed). For phlegm masses, oyster shell may be added; for wind-phlegm-fire disorder (which tends to cause spasms or paralysis), silkworm is often added; for thickened phlegm associated with yin deficiency, ophiopogon is often added; when food accumulation leads to phlegm production, shen-chu, malt, and crataegus may be included; schizandra is included in some formulas to astringe excess fluid production, but is in other formulas to help generate fluid when there is yin deficiency yielding insufficient mucus production.

Resolving Hot Phlegm

The herbs that resolve hot phlegm generally have a cold property; those with a salty or bitter taste are often used for resolving swellings, including tumors, while those with a sweet taste moisten dryness.

- Bamboo refers to the shavings of the stem of several species of bamboos, most commonly Phyllostachys nigra. The Chinese name, zhuru, means the edible part of the well-known plant called zhu. It has a sweet taste and a mild cold nature, entering the lung and stomach meridians to resolve thick phlegm and to control vomiting due to heat and accumulation in the stomach. It is an important ingredient of Aurantium and Bamboo Combination (Jupi Zhuru Tang) used for nausea, hiccoughing, and vomiting. The active components, including triterpenes, resolve thickened phlegm and reduce inflammation of the stomach.

Aurantium and Bamboo Combination		
Jupi Zhuru Tang		
Aurantium	Jupi; or use chenpi	12 g
Bamboo	Zhuru	12 g
Ginger	Shengjiang	9 g
Jujube	Dazao	5 pieces
Licorice	Zhi gancao	6 g

- Bamboo sap, in liquid form is called zhuli, and dried bamboo sap is often called tianzhuhuang (heavenly bamboo yellow); these materials have similar applications to bamboo shavings (zhuru), but are more cooling in nature (perhaps due to the higher content of minerals). These sap materials enter the heart meridian and treat phlegm mist obstructing the heart orifices, to relieve convulsions, paralysis, and high fever. Bamboo sap is included in patent medicines for phlegm-fire disorder, such as Baoying Dan, used for fever and difficult respiration due to acute ailment in infants.

Zhu Po Baoying Dan		
Patent remedy from Guangzhou		
Snake gallbladder	Sanshedan	12.9%
Scorpion	Quanxie	9.7%
Gastrodia	Tianma	8.0%
Silkworm	Jiangcan	8.0%
Siler	Fangfeng	8.0%
Uncaria	Gouteng	8.0%
Succinum	Hupo	7.2%
Bamboo sap	Tianzhuhuang	5.7%
Calomel	Qingfen	5.7%
Borneol	Bingpian	5.7%
Cicada	Chantui	5.7%
Pearl	Zhenzhu	5.4%
Musk	Shexiang	4.3%

- Clam shells are obtained from many species of bivalves, but especially Cyclina sinensis. The Chinese name, haigeke, simply refers to the ocean, hai, the clam, ge, and its shell, ke. Like other sea shells, it has a salty taste, a cold nature, and it influences the liver and lungs. It resolves phlegm masses, which include tenacious sputum in the lungs, and swellings. Clam shell is a major component of Isatis and Hai-ko Formula (Dai Ge San), comprised of those two herbs alone, for stubborn phlegm in the lungs that is discolored (due to toxic heat; an infection); it is also a major component of Atractylodes and Hai-ko Formula (Kaiyu Zhengyuan San) that is used for abdominal masses, such as uterine fibroids (this formula is a modification of Kaiyu Erchen Tang), which develop secondary to qi stagnation and food stagnation with phlegm accumulation. The active components of the clam shell are calcium salts and proteins.

Atractylodes and Hai-ko Formula		
Kaiyu Zhengyuan San		
Atractylodes	Baizhu	3 g
Citrus	Chenpi	3 g
Blue citrus	Qingpi	2 g
Cyperus	Xiangfuzi	3 g
Crataegus	Shanzha	3 g
Hai-ko	Haige	3 g
Platycodon	Jiegeng	3 g
Hoelen	Fuling	3 g
Cardamon	Sharen	1.5 g
Corydalis	Yansuhuo	3 g
Malt	Guya	3 g
Licorice	Gancao	1.5 g
Shen-chu	Shenqu	3 g
Ginger	Shengjiang	2 slices

- Bulbifera refers to the rhizome of Dioscorea bulbifera, one of several Dioscorea species used in Chinese medicine. The Chinese name huangyaozi refers to its yellow color and to the bulbous underground stem, with zi indicating offspring, as it does for aconite branch roots, fuzi. Its influence is cooling, affecting the liver and heart to reduce swellings associated with interior heat, such as carbuncles, lung abscess, breast lumps, goiter, and tumors. Bulbifera is a component of Jia Kang Wan for treating hyperthyroidism: it is one of several phlegm-resolving herbs used to remove the thyroid mass, which is interpreted as a phlegm mass. Researchers caution, however, that high dosage or prolonged use of bulbifera can cause liver damage. This herb is usually not used in by Western practitioners due to the safety concerns, though the amount in this formula is small and, thus, it is considered by Chinese physicians to be a safe level for use in China. Li Shizhen had written that bulbifera is "bitter in taste, mild in nature, and nonpoisonous, reducing heat by cooling the blood and curing goiter through removing toxins."

Jia Kang Wan		
(Main ingredients of pill used in clinical trial for hyperthyroid disease)		
Prunella	Xiakucao	16%
Oyster shell	Muli	12%
Sargassum	Haizao	12%
Laminaria	Kunbu	12%
Pinellia	Banxia	12%
Fritillaria	Zhebaimu	12%
Hoelen	Fuling	12%
Aurantium	Juhong	8%
Bulbifera	Huangyaozi	4%

- Cynanchum refers to the rhizome of Cynanchum stauntoni and related species. The Chinese name, baiqian, means white front, referring to the appearance of the leaves. The taste is acrid and sweet, and the influence is mildly cold. It enters the lung meridian to help moisten the lungs, aid the descent of qi, and expel profuse sputum. Cynanchum is a major ingredient of the Platycodon and Schizonepeta Formula (Zhi Sou San) used for the treatment of cough with excessive sputum. The active components are saponins that thin the sputum and relieve inflammation.

Platycodon and Schizonepeta Formula		
Zhi Sou San		
Cynanchum	Baiqian	17%
Platycodon	Jiegeng	17%
Schizonepeta	Jingjie	17%
Aster	Ziyuan	17%
Stemona	Baibu	17%
Citrus	Chenpi	9%
Licorice	Gancao	6%

- Fritillaria refers to two major species of fritillaria, F. cirrosa and F. thunbergii, members of the Lily family. Both varieties are bitter, mildly cold, and affect the lung and heart. The two species have similar actions and uses, but the cirrhosa species is deemed more suitable for moistening the lungs when there is a heat syndrome, and thunbergii is more suited for removing phlegm masses, including tumors. The Chinese name, beimu, makes reference to the appearance of the white bulbs like cowry shells (the cirrosa species is known as chuanbeimu because it comes from Sichuan Province; the thunbergii species is known as zhebeimu, produced in Zhejiang Province). In most formulas, the variety of fritillaria is not specified and, because it is more readily available and less expensive, zhebeimu is usually selected. Fritillaria is an important ingredient of Platycodon and Fritillaria Combination (Qingfei Tang), a traditional prescription for bronchitis that is mostly used in Japan. The formula nourishes yin and clears heat, two properties common to the lily bulbs, and the complex formulation is aimed at treating sputum that is sticky but profuse. The active components of fritillaria are steroidal alkaloids which have sedative, anti-inflammatory, and phlegm resolving actions.

Platycodon and Fritillaria Combination		
Qingfei Tang		
Platycodon	Jiegeng	6 g
Fritillaria	Beimu	6 g
Scute	Huangqin	6 g
Apricot seed	Xingren	6 g
Bamboo	Zhuru	6 g
Ophiopogon	Maimendong	9 g
Gardenia	Zhizi	6 g
Citrus	Chenpi	6 g
Hoelen	Fuling	9 g
Morus	Sangbaipi	6 g
Asparagus	tianmendong	6 g
Tang-kuei	Danggui	9 g
Jujube	Dazao	6 pieces
Fresh ginger	Shengjiang	1 slice
Licorice	Gancao	3 g
Schizandra	Wuweizi	1.5 g

- Lapis is a mineral which is well-known as a semi-precious stone laced with mica schist; in fact, today, Chinese doctors use the less expensive mica (which has a golden color) alone. The Chinese name, jinmengshi, refers to the inconsistent color meng, of the stone, shi, for which the golden variety, jin, has been selected. The taste is acrid and salty, and it has a cold nature. Lapis affects the lung and liver, resolving phlegm and calming agitation. Lapis is an ingredient in the Lapis and Scute Formula (Mengshi Guntan Wan) used for phlegm fire syndrome, as applied in the treatment of mental disorders, convulsions and tenacious sputum associated with an inflammatory disease, such as gastritis, bronchitis, pharyngitis, and tuberculosis.

Lapis and Scute Formula		
Mengshi Guntan Wan		
Lapis	Mengshi	35%
Rhubarb	Dahuang	26%
Scute	Huangqin	26%
Aquilaria	Chenxiang	13%

- Peucedanum refers to the roots of Peucedanum praeruptorum, a close relative of the more commonly used herb bupleurum. Its Chinese name, qianhu, reflects its comparison to bupleurum, called chaihu. The taste is bitter and acrid, it has a mild, cold nature and affects the lungs to resolve phlegm and to relieve coughing. It is especially used in cases of acute bronchitis, and because of its mild nature, it is used for both hot and cold syndromes. It is an important ingredient in the Perilla Fruit Combination (Suzi Jiangqi Tang), used for treatment of asthma, bronchitis, emphysema, and other lung disorders, given when there is copious sputum. The active components include flavonoids, such as peupraerin, which dilate the blood vessels and aid expectoration.

Perilla Fruit Combination		
Suzi Jiangqi Tang		
Perilla seed	Suzi	9 g
Pinellia	Banxia	9 g
Tang-kuei	Danggui	9 g
Peucedanum	Qianhu	6 g
Magnolia bark	Houpo	6 g
Cinnamon bark	Rougui	6 g
Licorice	Zhi gancao	6 g
Ginger	Shengjiang	3 slices

- Pumice refers to volcanic lava that has entered the ocean, becoming light due to the influence of steaming water, making it porous as it cools. The pores become filled with tiny marine life. The resulting material is salty, mildly cold, and influences the lungs to remove phlegm masses; its mild nature makes it suitable for treatment of children's coughs. It is also used for resolving swellings, such as goiter, tumors, and scrofula. Pumice is not included as an ingredient among traditional formulas. It is included in the modern formula Laminaria 4 (Hai Lin Pian), used for phlegm masses and tenacious sputum in the lungs. The active components of pumice are silicon dioxide, a component also found in bamboo sap, plus the minerals common to sea materials such as clam shells, mainly calcium salts.

Laminaria 4		
Hai Lin Pian		
Laminaria	Kunbu	40%
Sargassum	Haizao	39%
Oyster shell	Muli	10%
Pumice	Haifushi	10%
Sinapis	Baijiezi	1%

- Sterculia refers to the seed of Sterculia scahigera. Its Chinese name pangdahai, refers to the fact that the herb swells up when dipped in water and floats like a sponge. Although listed in the phlegm-resolving section of most Chinese herb texts, it has minimal direct action on phlegm, mainly having an "opening" action that aids the normal flow of mucus. It has a sweet taste and cold property, affecting the lungs and large intestine-moistening dryness, opening the lungs and throat, and promoting bowel movements. The herb is rarely included in traditional formulas, but it is sometimes used in modern clinical practice. For example is an ingredient of Yanhou Tang, used for the treatment of chronic pharyngitis. The active components of this herb have not yet been ascertained.

Yanhou Tang	
Lonicera	Jinyinhua
Ophiopogon	Maimendong
Chyrsanthemum	Juhua
Platycodon	Jiegeng
Sterculia	Pangdahai
Oroxylum	Muhudie
Licorice	Gancao

- Trichosanthes refers to a starchy root obtained from the Chinese gourd plant Trichosanthes kirilowii. The Chinese name, gualougen, simply refers to the root, gen, of the gourd; it is also called tianhuafen, indicating the white powder obtained from the root. The taste is sweet and sour and it has a cold property. It influences the lung and stomach, moistening dryness and clearing heat and swelling. It is most commonly used for diseases with thirst as a symptom, including diabetes. It is an important ingredient of Ophiopogon and Trichosanthes Combination (Maimendong Yin Zi), a formula used for diabetes and chronic bronchitis with dry cough. The active components of trichosanthes include sterols and saponins. The root is also the source of a protein drug, trichosanthin, commonly called Compound Q, which has been used as an abortifacient, a treatment for cancer, and a trial drug in the treatment of AIDS.

Ophiopogon and Trichosanthes Combination		
Maimendong Yin Zi		
Ophiopogon	Maimendong	21 g
Hoelen	Fuling	18 g
Rehmannia	Shengdi	12 g
Anemarrhena	Zhimu	9 g
Pueraria	Gegen	9 g
Trichosanthes root	Gualougen	6 g
Ginseng	Renshen	6 g
Bamboo	Zhuru	3 g
Schizandra	Wuweizi	3 g
Licorice	Gancao	3 g

- Trichosanthes seed is derived from the same plant as the root. The Chinese name, gualouren simply indicates that it is the seed of the gourd. The taste is bitter and it affects the lung and stomach as well as the large intestine to resolve phlegm and treat dryness. Trichosanthes seed is an ingredient of Anemarrhena and Fritillaria Formula (Ermu Ningsou Wan), a pill used for severe coughing with dryness. The active components include fatty acids and saponins. The whole trichosanthes gourd or just the outer portion are also used in Chinese medicine, with similar applications, especially used for treating persistent discharge of colored phlegm; the seed is selected in cases of congestion accompanied by constipation, while the outer portion is selected when there is sticky phlegm in the chest.

Anemarrhena and Fritillaria Formula		
Ermu Ningsou Wan		
Anemarrhena	Zhimu	10%
Fritillaria	Chuanbeimu	8%
Trichosanthes seed	Gualouren	10%
Morus bark	Sangbaipi	10%
Citrus	Chenpi	10%
Hoelen	Fuling	10%
Gardenia	Zhizi	10%
Scute	Huangqin	10%
Chih-shih	Zhishi	8%
Schizandra	Wuweizi	8%
Licorice	Gancao	6%

- Trichosanthes fruit is derived from the same plant as the root. The Chinese name, gualou simply indicates that it is this particular gourd. Sometimes, only the peel of the fruit is used; it is known as gualoupi. The taste is sweet and it affects the lung and stomach as well as the large intestine to resolve thick phlegm and treat dryness. Trichosanthes fruit is a major component of Trichosanthes, Bakeri, and Pinellia Combination (Gualou Xiebai Banxia Tang) which is used for phlegm accumulation in the chest area, affecting the heart and lungs, as occurs with some heart disease.

Trichosanthes, Bakeri, and Pinellia Combination		
Gualou Xiebai Banxia Tang		
Trichosanthes fruit	Gualou	3 g
Bakeri	Xiebai	4.5 g
Pinellia	Banxia	6 g

- Usnea refers to the parasitic plant Usnea longissima and related species, found growing from the branches of pine trees. The Chinese name, songluo, refers to its beard-like appearance on the pine tree. It has a bitter and sweet taste, cleanses the lungs, controls bleeding, and reduces inflammation and infection. It is an ingredient of Pinellia and Usnea Formula (Ying Jie San), used in the treatment of tumors that are comprised of a phlegm mass, such as melanomas and lymphatic tumors. The active components of usnea include usnic acid.

Pinellia and Usnea Formula		
Ying Jie San		
Fried wheat	Zhi Xiaomai	12 g
Usnea	Songluo	9 g
Pinellia	Banxia	9 g
Fritillaria	Zhebeimu	9 g
Sargassum	Haizao	9 g
Laminaria	Kunbu	9 g
Gentiana	Longdancao	9 g
Arca shells	Walengzi	9 g
Tetrapanax	Tongcao	9 g
Alum	Mingfan	9 g

- Laminaria refers to at least two seaweeds, Laminaria japonica or Ecklonia kurome, the latter being the most common source in modern times. The Chinese name kunbu refers to the appearance of its many broad leaves. The seaweed, like others, is salty in taste and has a cold property. It influences the liver, kidney, and stomach, reducing swellings and eliminating excess moisture. Since laminaria is almost always combined with another seaweed, sargassum, a representative formula using laminaria is presented with the sargassum entry. The salts in seaweed may be responsible for both diuretic and phlegm-resolving activities. There are also polysaccharides that reduce lung irritation. Laminaria is mainly used in formulas that "soften" masses, being used for ovarian cysts, thyroid swellings, and tumors.

- Sargassum is a seaweed obtained from Sargassum fusiforme and some related species. The Chinese name, haizao simply means sea hair. Its taste is salty and bitter, and it has a cold nature. It influences the liver, kidney, and stomach to treat swelling, edema, and phlegm accumulation. Its properties are like those of laminaria, with which it is usually combined. Sargassum and laminaria are ingredients of the Sargassum and Laminaria Combination, sometimes called the Seaweed Combination (Haizao Yuhu Tang). It is used in the treatment of thyroid swellings and tumors.

Sargassum and Tu-huo Combination		
Haizao Yuhu Tang		
Sargassum	Haizao	3 g
Laminaria	Kunbu	3 g
Pinellia	Banxia	3 g
Citrus	Chenpi	3 g
Blue citrus	Qingpi	3 g
Forsythia	Lianqiao	3 g
Fritillaria	Zhebeimu	3 g
Tang-kuei	Danggui	3 g
Cnidium	Chuanxiong	3 g
Tu-huo	Duhuo	3 g
Licorice	Gancao	3 g
Kelp	Haidai	1.5 g

- Chu-dan is the bile obtained from pigs; the Chinese name zhudan simply refers to the pig's (zhu) gallbladder or bile (dan). It has a bitter taste and affects the lung, liver, and gallbladder. Chu-dan is used to treat cough with profuse phlegm or difficult expectoration due to a lung heat syndrome; it is also utilized for a wide range of heat syndromes, including swollen and painful eyes, sore throat, dysentery, boils, inflammation of the liver, and congestion of the bile duct or gallbladder. It is an ingredient of cough syrups, such as Chuan Ke Ling, and is often used as an inexpensive substitute for snake bile (shedan). The active constituents are bile acids.

Chuan Ke Ling		
(patent cough syrup)		
Platycodon	Jiegeng	35%
Licorice	Gancao	30%
Apricot seed	Xingren	25%
Chu-dan	Zhudan	10%

Herbs for Cold Phlegm

- Arisaema refers to the processed tuber of Arisaema consanguineum. The Chinese name tiannanxing means heaven's southern star. It is acrid and bitter, and somewhat toxic before processing, usually with pig's bile (it is then often called dannanxing; dan means gallbladder or bile). Its influence is mainly on the lung, liver, and spleen, resolving phlegm, calming wind, and drying dampness; it is also used to resolve resulting heart phlegm congestion, for stroke, paralysis, and convulsion. Arisaema is a major ingredient of the Pinellia and Arisaema Combination (Qingshi Huatan Tang), used for pain and numbness due to phlegm obstruction of the nerves, muscles, and joints. The main active components are saponins that thin the phlegm and reduce inflammation.

Pinellia and Arisaema Combination		
Qingshi Huatan Tang		
Pinellia	Banxia	12 g
Hoelen	Fuling	12 g
Atractylodes	Baizhu	12 g
Arisaema	Tiannanxing	9 g
Scute	Huangqin	9 g
Fresh ginger	Shengjiang	3 slices
Citrus	Chenpi	7.5 g
Sinapis	Baijiezi	4.5 g
Bamboo sap	Tianjuhuang	4.5 g
Chiang-huo	Qianghuo	4.5 g
Angelica	Baizhi	4.5 g
Licorice	Gancao	4.5 g

- Centipeda refers to the whole plant of Centipeda minima, a member of the Dandelion Family; it should not be confused with the insect centipede, which is also used in Chinese medicine. One of the Chinese names, shihusui, makes reference to similarities in its appearance to husui, coriander; it is more commonly know as ebushicao ("herb that even a goose won't eat" because of its strong taste). It has an acrid taste and is said to enter the lung meridian because of its strong effects on the lungs and sinuses, alleviating stuffiness. In addition, it clarifies obstructed vision and can be used in treating infections of the respiratory system or intestines. It is not commonly included in traditional Chinese formulas, but is used in some modern clinical applications. It is an ingredient of the formula Xanthium 12, devised in the U.S. to treat allergy reactions, especially sinus allergies. The active components of centipeda include taraxesterols found also in dandelion, and flavonoids that reduce allergy reaction.

Xanthium 12		
Kang Xieqi Pian		
Xanthium	Cangerzi	13%
Sophora	Kushen	12%
Bupleurum	Chaihu	9%
Centipeda	Ebushicao	9%
Scute	Huangqin	9%
Cynanchum	Baiqian	9%
Siler	Fangfeng	8%
Mume	Wumei	8%
Ginseng	Renshen	6%
Licorice	Gancao	6%
Asarum	Xixin	6%
Schizandra	Wuweizi	5%

- Gleditsia refers to the sharp spines of Gleditsia officinalis and related species of the member of the Legume family. The Chinese name, zaoci, simply refers to the spike, ci, of the plant commonly called zao, meaning black, because black soap was made from the saponins of the fruits. It has an acrid taste and a mild warm quality. It enters the lung meridian and aids in dispersing phlegm masses. Gleditsia is an ingredient in many antitumor formulas, such as Angelica and Mastic Combination (Xianfang Huoming Yin), used for carbuncles, abscess, swelling ulcers, and tumors. The main active components are saponins. Gleditsia fruits (zaojia) have similar properties, but are mainly used for cases of phlegm obstruction of the orifices, thus treating stroke, convulsion, and paralysis.

Angelica and Mastic Combination		
Xianfang Huoming Yin		
Lonicera	Jinyinhua	9 g
Citrus	Chenpi	9 g
Anteater scales	Chuanshanjia	3 g
Angelica	Baizhi	3 g
Gleditsia spine	Zaoci	3 g
Trichosanthes root	Gualuogen	3 g
Peony	Baishao	3 g
Myrrh	Moyao	3 g
Frankincense	Ruxiang	3 g
Fritillaria	Zhebeimu	3 g
Tang-kuei	Danggui	3 g
Siler	Fangfeng	3 g
Licorice	Gancao	3 g

- Inula refers to the flowers of Inula britannica, an internationally used herb of the Dandelion family. Its name xuanfuhua, refers to the dense curled shape of the flower head. The taste is acrid and bitter, and its property is mildly warm. It affects the lung and large intestine, and the spleen and stomach, resolving phlegm, causing qi to descend, and softening hardness. Inula is an ingredient of the Schizonepeta and Pinellia Formula (Qingfei Cao San) used for the treatment of bronchitis with productive cough and sinus congestion. The active components are mainly taraxasterol and related compounds that reduce inflammation and disperse phlegm.

Schizonepeta and Pinellia Formula		
Qingfei Cao San		
Schizonepeta	Jingjie	17.5 g
Peucedanum	Qianhu	13.5 g
Inula	Xuanfuhua	9 g
Asarum	Xixin	9 g
Hoelen	Fuling	5.4 g
Pinellia	Banxia	4.5 g
Licorice	Gancao	3 g
Ginger	Shengjiang	2 slices
Jujube	Dazao	3 pieces

- Pinellia refers to the processed tuber of Pinellia ternata, the most frequently used of all the phlegm-resolving herbs. The Chinese name, banxia, means half summer, and refers to the fact that it is collected in mid-summer. It has an acrid taste and is toxic until processed, usually cooked with ginger juice. It enters the spleen and stomach meridians, harmonizing the stomach and reducing the production of phlegm due to undigested food and excessive upward movement of qi and moisture. It is the key herb of Pinellia Combination (Banxia Xiexin Tang), a formula that is widely used and often modified slightly for specific applications; it is mostly used for indigestion, nausea, vomiting, gastritis, and ulcer. The active components are many, including alkaloids, phenols, and sterols, producing a sedative, antiemetic, and phlegm-resolving action.

Pinellia Combination		
Banxia Xiexin Tang		
Pinellia	Banxia	18 g
Ginseng	Renshen	9 g
Jujube	Dazao	6 pieces
Fresh ginger	Shengjiang	3 slices
Coptis	Huanglian	3 g
Scute	Huangqin	9 g
Licorice	Zhi Gancao	9 g

- Platycodon refers to the roots of Platycodon graniflorum; it is a relative of the tonic herbs codonopsis and adenophora. The Chinese name, jiegeng, makes reference to the quality of the plant's stalk. Its taste is acrid and bitter, and its property is neutral. It enters the lung meridian to ventilate the lungs, resolve phlegm and disperse cold; because of its neutral quality, however, it is frequently used in treatment of lung heat and sore throat. It is an ingredient of the Fritillaria and Platycodon Formula (Ning Sou Wan), a pill that is used for acute and chronic bronchitis with persisting cough and excessive sputum. The active components of platycodon are saponins, sterols, and triterpenoids, that reduce inflammation and thin the sputum.

Fritillaria and Platycodon Formula		
Ning Sou Wan		
Platycodon	Jiegeng	10%
Perilla fruit	Zisuzi	10%
Dendrobium	Shihu	10%
Fritillaria	Beimu	10%
Hoelen	Fuling	10%
Pinellia	Banxia	10%
Mentha	Bohe	8%
Morus	Sangbaipi	8%
Apricot seed	Xingren	8%
Red citrus	Juhong	6%
Wheat sprout	Xiaomai	6%
Licorice	Gancao	4%

- Sinapis, sometimes called brassica, refers to the seed of Brassica alba, also called Sinapis alba, and related species of mustard. The Chinese name, baijiezi, refers to the white seed that confers strength. It has an acrid taste and enters the lung meridian to promote the flow of qi in the chest, expel phlegm, and disperse swellings. Sinapis is an ingredient in Lige Huotan Tang, used for the treatment of phlegm accumulation that leads to hiccups, choking sensation, and difficulty consuming food. Even though sinapis is warming, it is included in this formula for phlegm stagnation that has turned hot, because of its powerful dispersing qualities, counterbalanced by inclusion of coptis, gardenia, and gypsum. The active components of sinapis include the glycoside sinalbin, which has expectorant properties.

Lige Huotan Tang		
Pinellia	Banxia	9 g
Red citrus	Juhong	9 g
Chih-shih	Zhishi	9 g
Areca seed	Binglang	9 g
Aquilaria	Chenxiang	9 g

Platycodon	Jiegeng	9 g
Trichosanthes root	Gualougen	9 g
Coptis	Haunglian	9 g
Gardenia	Zhizi	9 g
Cyperus	Xiangfuzi	9 g
Sinapis	Baijiezi	6 g
Gypsum	Shigao	12 g
Tea	Xicha	3 g

- Typhonium, often called "white aconite," is obtained either from the tuber of Typhonium giganteum or Aconitum koreanum. The Chinese name, baifuzi, means white aconite. The taste is acrid and sweet, and it affects mainly the stomach, to get rid of phlegm that rises due to adverse movement of qi. The herb is used for phlegm obstruction causing paralysis, pain, or convulsion. Typhonium is an important ingredient of the formula True Jade Powder (Yu Zhen San) used for tonic muscular paralysis. The active components of the Typhonium species are sterols while the Aconitum species yield alkaloids, the latter having a stronger pain-relieving action.

True Jade Powder		
Yu Zhen San		
Typhonium	Baifuzi	3 g
Arisaema	Tiannanxing	3 g
Siler	Fangfeng	3 g
Angelica	Baizhi	3 g
Gastrodia	Tianma	3 g
Chiang-huo	Qianghuo	3 g

References

- Chinese-herbology, entry: newworldencyclopedia.org, Retrieved 3 June, 2019

- Chinese-herbal-therapy, guides, wellness, org, scassets: clevelandclinic.org, Retrieved 17 May, 2019

- Complementary-therapies/traditional-chinese-herbal-remedies, diagnosis-and-treatment, cancer-information: cancer.ca, Retrieved 13 February, 2019

- Herbs-that-release-the-exterior: clinicalgate.com, Retrieved 29 March, 2019

- Herbs-that-warm-the-interior-and-expel-cold-cold-hands-and-feet-fear-of-cold-pale-complexion-no-thirst-desire-for-warm: holosapiens.com, Retrieved 26 July, 2019

- Herbs-that-regulate-the-energy, materia-medica: holosapiens.com, Retrieved 29 June, 2019

Chapter 4
Acupuncture and Moxibustion

The branch of traditional Chinese medicine which involves the insertion of needles into the body is termed as acupuncture. Moxibustion refers to a form of therapy within Chinese traditional medicine where dried mugwort is burned on specific point of the body. The topics elaborated in this chapter will help in gaining a better perspective about moxibustion as well as the different practices within acupuncture such as auricular acupuncture and electroacupuncture.

Acupuncture

Acupuncture is the insertion of very fine, filiform needles through the skin at specific points on the body with the intention of manipulating Qi. The filiform needles are solid, as opposed to the hollow hypodermic needles most people are familiar with, and are usually made of stainless steel, but can also be gold or silver.

Flow of Qi through the Body

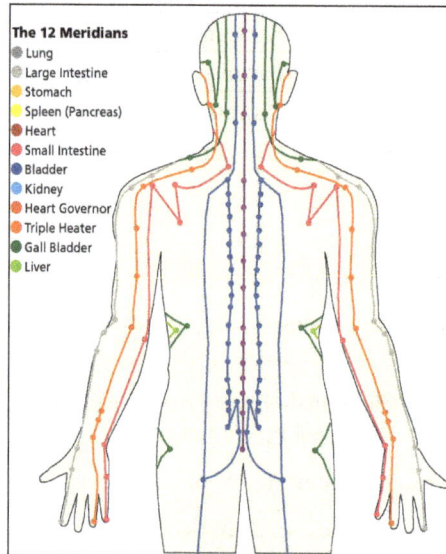

Acupuncture is based upon the jing luo channel network theory of the circulation of Qi. Although Qi permeates every part of the body, it tends to collect and travel along channels called "jing luo." These are the so-called "meridians" of acupuncture. The jing luo channel system connects all aspects of the body together into one network of energetic communication.

Just as water flowing through a landscape tends to seek the path of least resistance, so Qi flows through the body. The flow of Qi follows the folds and creases of the body's landscape. It follows the divisions between muscles and the clefts between muscles and bones, collecting in the small hollows and depressions of the body to form pools of Qi.

These "pools of Qi" are places where Qi is concentrated and more accessible. They are the acupuncture points, where Qi can be accessed and manipulated through the use of finger pressure (acupressure), massage techniques (tui na; literally "pinch and pull"), dermal friction (gua sha), cupping, moxibustion (a form of heat therapy), and, of course, acupuncture.

Uses of Acupuncture

TCM practitioners use acupuncture to treat a wide range of conditions. Some of the conditions for which acupuncture is commonly used include:

- Pain,
- Injury,
- Trauma,
- Repetitive strain conditions like tennis elbows and carpal tunnel syndrome,
- Headache,
- Rheumatoid and osteoarthritis,
- Back pain and sciatica,
- Fibromyalgia,
- Dysmenorrhea and other gynecological conditions,
- Asthma,
- Post operative and chemotherapy nausea,
- Stroke rehabilitation,
- Patients undergoing recovery from addiction and substance abuse.

Side Effects of Acupuncture

Side effects are rare. Patients may occasionally experience slight bruising at the point of needle insertion.

Needle Shock: A feeling of faintness, chilliness and perhaps slight nausea. Needle shock happens rarely, but when it does, it is most likely to happen in situations in which the patient is very nervous about the needles, is extremely exhausted or fatigued, or is experiencing low blood sugar from not having eaten for a long period of time before the acupuncture treatment.

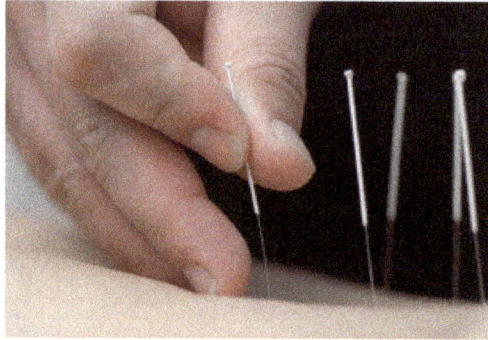

Needle shock can be disquieting to the patient but is not considered harmful. Most states that regulate acupuncture require practitioners to provide informed consent forms outlining these possible side-effects.

When shouldn't Acupuncture be used?

The use of acupuncture is not as prominent or may even be contraindicated in the treatment of:

- Infants and very young children;

- Very weak or very elderly patients;

- People with compromised immunity;

- Patients suffering with certain bleeding disorders or severe blood loss;

- Patients who are very weak, emaciated, who are suffering from low blood sugar, or who have collapsed due to fatigue and exhaustion;

- Patients with significantly low blood pressure;

- Patients who are suffering with extreme anxiety or who are very nervous about the needles;

- Pregnancy: While acupuncture is generally considered safe for most women during pregnancy, there are certain acupuncture points that are forbidden during pregnancy. Pregnant women should talk with their OB-GYN doctor and their TCM practitioner about these restrictions and any other concerns regarding their pregnancy before undergoing an acupuncture treatment.

Types of Pain Treated by Acupuncture

Acupuncture is relatively cost-effective compared to other therapies and the risk of adverse effects is generally considered much lower than pharmacological treatments. 5 types of chronic pain that acupuncture may help to relieve.

Low Back Pain

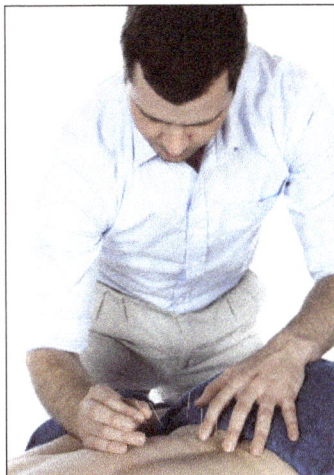

Back pain is one of the most common reasons that people seek acupuncture treatment, and studies on chronic low back pain have shown that the therapy can provide short-term relief and improve function. Some research has demonstrated that acupuncture can be more effective in relieving symptoms from acute low back pain than medications. Patients with nonspecific chronic low back pain have reported improvements in functional limitations with acupuncture. A common regimen for chronic low back pain is 11 25-minute sessions, performed twice a week.

Head, Face and Neck Pain

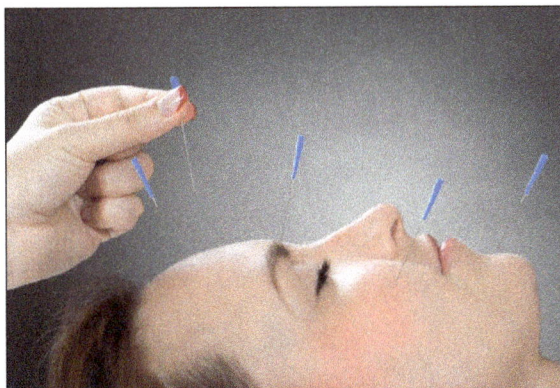

Several forms of head and facial pain, including pain caused by trigeminal neuralgia (pain along the trigeminal nerve which carries signals from the face to the brain) or tempromandibular joint (TMJ) dysfunction, can find relief with acupuncture. Treatment is most successful when the pain is neuromuscular rather than the result of joint damage. Acupuncture can help to alleviate discomfort by targeting the source of the pain, such as around the ear and jaw, but may also include areas near the elbows, knees, and big toes, because of their meridian connections. Weekly 30-minute sessions are typical, and may be used in conjunction with jaw appliances, medications, or surgery depending on the severity of the pain and condition.

Osteoarthritis

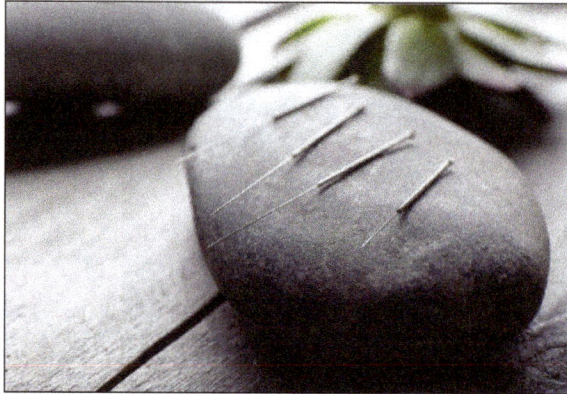

Many individuals with osteoarthritis (OA) are accustomed to mainstream medications and therapies to manage the debilitating effects of the condition but many also find relief in acupuncture when used in combination with those treatments. The placement of needles can trigger endorphins as well as the production of cortisol, an anti-inflammatory hormone. Research has shown that the flow of these chemicals can help to reduce pain sensation. Acupuncture appears most effective in OA of the knee and spine. Results are typically seen after three or more sessions and last about a month.

Fibromyalgia

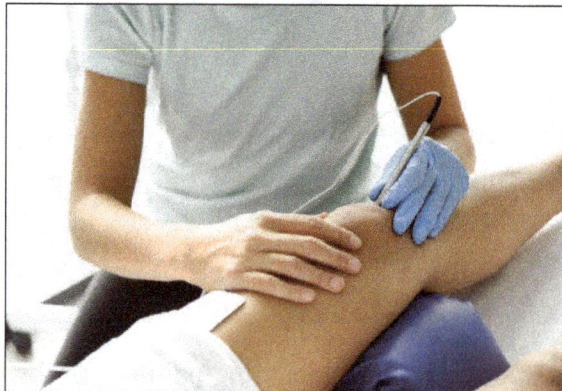

Individuals with fibromyalgia tend to experience pain in many areas of their body, and report accompanying symptoms such as joint stiffness, fatigue, and limited function.

Treatment options are limited to relieving pain and boosting physical ability. Acupuncture, however, can be used to enhance the effect of medication and therapies, contributing to the patient's overall well-being. Electrical stimulation, or electroacupuntre, has been shown to be more effective with fibromyalgia patients than needling alone. Sessions typically last 20 to 30 minutes and symptoms tend to improve within a few weeks.

Post-operative Pain

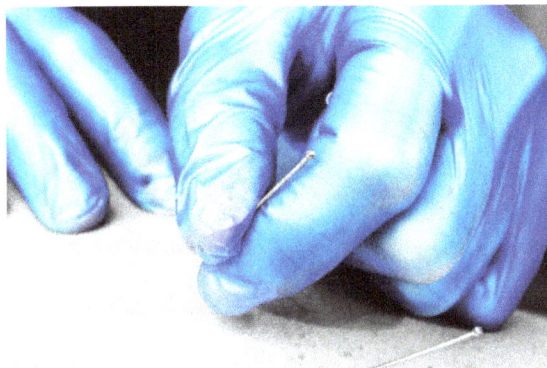

Traditional Chinese Medical sites a series of acupoints located near the spinal vertebrae, that when stimulated by acupuncture, can alleviate pain caused by a recent operation. Because access to these points may be limited during surgery, one option is to insert fine intradermal needles before an operation and keep them in position throughout the procedure as well as during recovery. This approach can help to reduce the need for opioid-based pain relief and associated side effects. It is believed that acupuncture can facilitate the release of neuropeptides in the central nervous system as well, leading to an analgesic, or pain-relieving, effect.

Auricular Acupuncture

Auricular acupuncture, also known as auricular therapy, auriculo-acupuncture and ear acupuncture is based on the principles of Traditional Chinese Medicine. Auricular therapy is widely used for many conditions, including addiction treatment, mood disorders, obesity, pain, and other conditions. This medical system emphasizes a holistic approach to medicine, an approach that treats the whole person. The acupuncture points found on the ear help to regulate the body's internal organs, structures, and functions.

Auricular therapy has a long history of use in China. It was mentioned in the most famous of ancient Chinese medical textbooks, "The Yellow Emperor's Classic of Internal Medicine." In modern times, auricular therapy has been shown to stimulate the release of endorphins, the body's own feel-good chemicals.

Uses of Ear Acupuncture in Treatment

Ear acupuncture is generally incorporated into a regular acupuncture treatment. In addition to using acupuncture points on the rest of the body, your acupuncturist may select a few ear acupuncture points that they feel will be helpful for your particular condition.

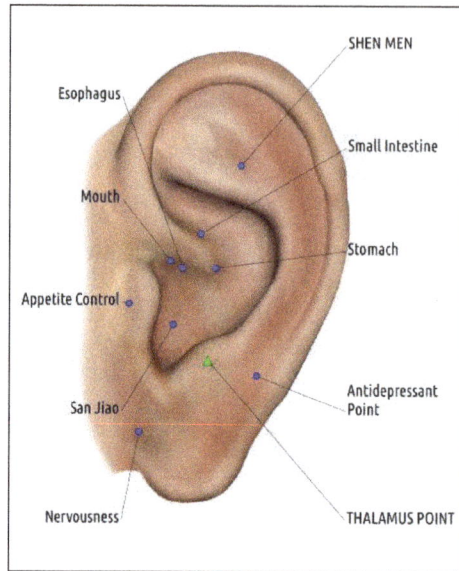

Ear Seeds and Ear Tacks

Ear acupuncture points may be stimulated for a longer period of time by using ear seeds or ear tacks. Ear seeds are small seeds from the Vaccaria plant. These seeds are held in place on the ear with a small piece of adhesive tape. Ear seeds may be left in the ear for a few days or up to two weeks. Ear tacks are very small needles with an adhesive backing. Ear tacks are inserted into the ear and left in the ear for a few days or up to one week.

Health Benefits of Ear Acupuncture

Although ear acupuncture is largely based on the principles of traditional Chinese medicine (a form of alternative medicine that originated in China), it was developed in the mid-20th century by French scientist Paul Nogier.

Uses

Ear acupuncture is used to improve the body's flow of vital energy (also known as chi or qi) and to restore a balance between yin and yang (two opposing but complementary energies) within the internal organs. In traditional Chinese medicine, each of these effects is considered essential in treating disease and achieving health.

In alternative medicine, ear acupuncture is typically used for these and other health conditions:

- Allergies

- Anxiety

- Arthritis

- Chronic pain

- Constipation

- Depression

- Fibromyalgia

- Headaches

- Insomnia

- Irritable bowel syndrome

- Low back pain

- Migraines

In addition, ear acupuncture is sometimes used to enhance mood, aid in smoking cessation, alleviate pain, promote sounder sleep, relieve stress, and support weight loss.

Benefits

Although large-scale clinical trials on ear acupuncture are currently lacking, a number of studies suggest that this therapy may aid in the treatment of a variety of health conditions.

Insomnia

Several studies indicate that ear acupuncture may help ease insomnia. These studies include a 2003 trial published in Complementary Therapies in Medicine, which tested the effects of a form of ear acupuncture that involves using magnetic pearls to stimulate acupuncture points.

For the study, 15 elderly people with insomnia were treated with ear acupuncture for three weeks. Results revealed that participants experienced a significant increase in both the quality and quantity of sleep, with improvements lasting for six months after treatment ended.

Smoking

So far, research on ear acupuncture's effectiveness as a smoking cessation aid has yielded mixed results. According to the study's authors, this success rate makes ear acupuncture "a competitive alternative to orthodox medicine withdrawal methods."

A trial involving 125 people found that ear acupuncture was no more effective than placebo treatment in improving the rate of smoking cessation. The study involved five consecutive weeks of once-a-week treatments.

Migraines

Ear acupuncture may be useful in the treatment of migraines. Analyzing findings on 35 migraine patients, the study's authors determined that two months of weekly ear acupuncture treatments led to significant improvements in pain and mood.

Post-surgery Pain

Investigators sized up 17 studies on ear acupuncture's effectiveness in pain management. The report's authors concluded that ear acupuncture may be effective for the treatment of a variety of types of pain, especially postoperative pain.

Constipation

Ear acupuncture may aid in the treatment of constipation. The authors, however, noted major flaws in the studies and recommend more research to confirm these findings.

Using Ear Acupuncture for Health

If you're considering trying ear acupuncture, make sure to consult your physician first. Self-treating and avoiding or delaying standard care can have serious consequences.

Electroacupuncture

Electroacupuncture is similar to acupuncture, a widely practiced form of traditional Chinese medicine (TCM). Acupuncture involves the use of thin needles to stimulate specific pressure points linked to unwanted symptoms.

In standard acupuncture, one needle is used at each treatment point. Electroacupuncture is a modified form that uses two needles.

A mild electric current passes between these needles during treatment. This current generally applies more stimulation to acupoints than needle twirling or other hand manipulation techniques an acupuncturist might use.

People use electroacupuncture to address a range of symptoms and health issues, including:

- Chemotherapy-related nausea

- Arthritis

- Pain

- Stress

- Addiction

- Tinnitus

Working

In TCM, your health depends on the flow of qi (energy) in your body. This energy travels along invisible pathways, known as meridians. These are found throughout your body.

Qi is believed to help keep your body in balance and promote its natural ability to heal itself. A blocked or disrupted flow of qi can negatively impact physical and emotional well-being.

That's where electroacupuncture comes in. It stimulates the points linked to your symptoms to help restart the flow of qi. Two needles are placed around the point while a machine delivers an electrical impulse to them. Electroacupuncture is intended to help increase the potential healing effects of standard acupuncture.

Procedure

Electroacupuncture is typically done by an acupuncturist. Here's what a session might look like:

- Your acupuncturist will evaluate your symptoms and select points for treatment.

- They'll insert a needle at the treatment point and another needle nearby.

- Once the needles are inserted to the correct depth, your acupuncturist will use electrodes to connect the needles to a special electroacupuncture machine.

- After the electrodes are attached, they'll turn on the machine. Electroacupuncture machines have adjustable current and voltage settings. Low voltages and frequencies will be used at first, though your acupuncturist may adjust the frequency and voltage of the current during treatment.

- The electric current pulsates, alternating between the two needles.

A typical session might last between 10 and 20 minutes, which is less than the average acupuncture session.

Effectiveness

Electroacupuncture is fairly new treatment, so there isn't much evidence to support its effectiveness for different uses. Still, a handful of studies suggest that it may provide some relief from chemotherapy side effects, arthritis, and acute (short-term) pain.

Arthritis

Looked at two studies exploring the benefits of acupuncture for rheumatoid arthritis (RA). One study used electroacupuncture treatments. In this study, those who received electroacupuncture treatment reported a significant reduction in knee pain just 24 hours after treatment. This effect lasts as long as four months after treatment.

However, note that the study included only a small number of participants and was of low quality. A study from 2017 looked at 11 randomized controlled trials on electroacupuncture for knee osteoarthritis. The results suggest electroacupuncture helped to both reduce pain and improve movement. The authors noted that the studies seemed to suggest four weeks of treatment were needed.

The study authors concluded by emphasizing the need for more high-quality trials to support electroacupuncture's treatment benefits.

Acute Pain

Looked at multiple preclinical animal studies on electroacupuncture's use as a form of pain relief. The results suggest that electroacupuncture can help to reduce different types of pain.

The authors also found evidence to suggest a combination of electroacupuncture and pain medication may be more effective than medication alone. This is promising, as it could mean that using electroacupuncture for pain relief may reduce the need for high doses of medicine.

Keep in mind that these results came from animal studies. More research is needed to understand the effects of electroacupuncture on pain in humans.

Chemotherapy-related Nausea

11 randomized trials looked at the use of acupuncture to reduce chemotherapy-related vomiting. The authors noted that electroacupuncture appeared to be more helpful for reducing vomiting right after a chemotherapy treatment than standard acupuncture.

Side Effects

As with standard acupuncture, electroacupuncture can cause a few side effects for certain people.

These might include:

- Mild nausea,

- Dizziness, feeling faint, or fainting,

- Pain or light bleeding when the needle is inserted,

- Redness or bruising at the needle site,

- Infection at the needle site, though this is rare when single-use sterile needles are used.

If the tingling or vibration of the electric current causes discomfort, tell your acupuncturist right away. If the voltage is too strong, the sensation could become unpleasant. Electric shock is possible, but it's rare if your acupuncturist is trained and the machine is working properly.

Risks Involved

Electroacupuncture is generally very safe if done by a skilled provider. However, if it isn't performed correctly, electroacupuncture can cause internal injuries or even electric shock.

In addition, you shouldn't try electroacupuncture if you:

- Are pregnant,

- Have heart disease,

- Have had a stroke,

- Have a pacemaker,

- Have epilepsy,

- Experience seizures.

It's generally recommended to talk to your doctor before trying a new treatment, especially if you have any underlying health issues.

Long-term Benefits of Acupuncture

Acupuncture is an alternative medical practice that has been enjoying more and more popularity in recent years. Acupuncture can help you by using your own body's natural abilities to heal.

Treatments are able to provide both short-term relief and long-term benefits. The process is simple and easy. Starting acupuncture today can provide the long-term benefits of acupuncture to you for years to come.

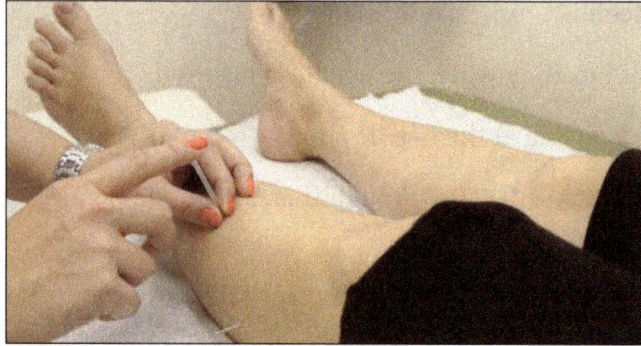

Acupuncture's Physical Benefits

The body reacts to injuries in different ways, most noticeably with an increase in chemical production and blood flow. The body receives a surge of useful chemicals, which move through your body's systems quickly with the increased blood flow. Different chemicals produced by your brain provide different benefits. Because the needles contain no chemicals, your body is using its own substances to heal. This means that acupuncture has no side effects.

The body's collagen production may also increase with acupuncture, which makes the skin smoother, erases wrinkles, and helps tone the face. Endorphins, which act as natural pain relievers, relax the muscles and help with chronic pain. Acupuncture affects natural processes in ways that ease physical issues and alleviate mental problems.

Mental Benefits of Acupuncture

Acupuncture treatments bring out the body's ability to benefit itself. Treatments can help with long-lasting and deep-seated disorders such as anxiety, depression, and insomnia. Acupuncture can ease pain and provide relief to disorders that cause discomfort. The body's more relaxed, comfortable state can do wonders for mental state and mood.

Emotional Stability through Acupuncture

Stress or other disorders may be the result of chemical imbalance or chronic pains racking the body. Acupuncture treatments spur the release and spread of positive brain chemicals throughout the body. The brain dictates what is missing and pushes certain natural processes to help restore balance.

The body's relaxed condition results in a more stable and comfortable emotional state. Acupuncture has the capacity to keep the body healthy, with its processes running smoothly through continued treatments.

Continuing Acupuncture Treatments for Long-term Benefits

Acupuncture treatments can help the body through pushing its natural processes to cause a natural, lasting change. Other treatments that involve chemicals or medication may put you at risk of side-effects. A drug chemical reaction gone badly is capable of even putting you in the hospital.

Acupuncture uses the body's natural healing ability for wellness and wellbeing. Repeated treatments not only continue to benefit you, but they occur without risk of side effects. You could see an increase in positive health benefits that may last a lifetime.

Reduces Chronic Pain

This is perhaps the most common and celebrated use of acupuncture on the human body, and as such, it has undergone the most research to test its validity. A recent study has shown acupuncture to reduce pain up to 15% when used for a variety of different types of pain, but primarily focused on chronic back pain that may result from physical stress, poor sleeping habits, old injuries that never fully healed, tightness of muscles, pregnancy, or other sources. Knee pain is another common affliction that causes people to try acupuncture, and although the studies have occasionally contradicted one another, there is a decent amount of positive research results that make acupuncture a legitimate way to reduce knee pain from surgery, or from the pain associated with osteoarthritis and aging. A study showed that patients with chronic knee pain showed short and long term benefits over those patients who either received sham acupuncture or not acupuncture at all, so there must be something positive going on in this traditional style or pain management.

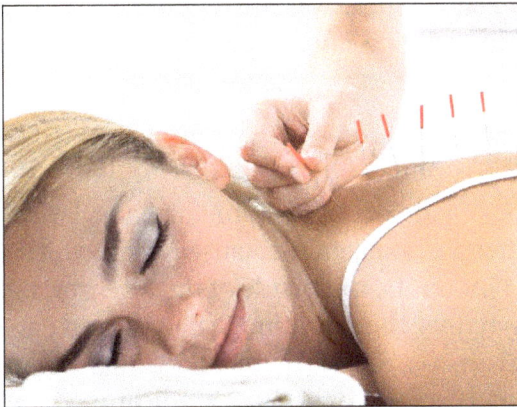

Reduces the Risk of Arthritis

Arthritis can be a debilitating disease that affects tens of millions of people around the world. Unfortunately, the benefits of modern medicine often fall short in fixing it over the long term, which means you must constantly (at least once daily) take powerful medicine to relieve the joint pain. Acupuncture offers a different option for reducing the painful and debilitating effects of arthritis. In the traditional belief system of acupuncture, there are 14 meridians, or energy channels, in the body that allow for the flow of qi, or natural body energy. These meridians often correspond to key nerve endings throughout the body that act as receptors for impulses from parts of the body like our knees, back, joints, temples, facial muscles, etc.

By inserting needles onto these meridians, our nerve endings communicate with our brains, and tell it that our muscles feel aching or "full". This will cause the release of endorphins, which are typically released during stress for an energy boost and to block pain receptors. These endorphins, combined with the normal neurotransmitters that affect nerve impulses, may be able to stop the pain associated with arthritis that physically limits so many people. One very unusual form of acupuncture that is gaining ground is called BVA (Bee Venom Acupuncture) where bee venom is topically applied to an acupuncture point of penetration. Studies have shown positive results between this style of acupuncture and a reduction in pain associated with arthritis.

Relieves Migraines

Another of the most popular applications of acupuncture in recent years has been for the relief of migraines and headaches, both in terms of pain relief and reduction in frequency. Although the exact mechanism to prevent these conditions via acupuncture around the face, neck, and scalp is not fully understood, positive results from research have in some ways justified, dozens of generations of this treatment method.

Neck pain has actually been one of the most highly verified and proven conditions for which acupuncture is effective. There was nearly unanimous support and proof of acupuncture being a reliable and side-effect free way to relieve chronic neck pain, very often the pain that can lead to constantly tense muscles, soreness, and headaches.

Prevents Nausea and Vomiting

Along with strong proof in support of acupuncture alleviating neck pain, it has also been shown as a very effective tool against nausea and vomiting. There is a particular acupuncture pressure point on the underside of the forearm, near the wrist, that when stimulated, is thought to reduce the sensation of nausea that can induce vomiting. After surgery, when a patient is recovering from the effects of anesthesia, they very often experience postoperative nausea and vomiting. A study argued that acupuncture was just as effective as antiemetic drugs that are commonly given to recovering patients. And again, the side effects of antiemetic drugs can change your body chemistry, something that most people who employ acupuncture try to avoid.

Chemotherapy is often used as a treatment option for cancer patients, and it can be a very effective way of saving lives. However, the side effects of chemotherapy are quite severe and include hair loss, nausea, and vomiting, among others. Another study showed that acupuncture was effective in preventing nausea and vomiting on the day of the chemotherapy, however, it did not that the acupuncture did not stop immediate nausea following the treatment, or delayed nausea in the following days.

Manages Anxiety

There have been a number of studies done on the effects of acupuncture on anxiety, including generalized anxiety disorder, anxiety neurosis, and perioperative anxiety. Like many of the other uses of acupuncture, the exact mechanism is not completely understood, but clinical trials show a positive correlation between anxiety reduction and acupuncture. Furthermore, when acupuncture was added to a pharmaceutical regimen for the management of stress and anxiety, and the medical dosage is decreased, results were actually better than when acupuncture was not involved. On top of that, the side effects of anti-anxiety drugs can be very intense, including nausea, mood swings, and depression, so any reduction of dosage without a return of the anxiety should be seen as a smart choice.

Reduces Insomnia

Studies have shown that acupuncture can reduce the frequency of insomnia for many people. It shows that acupuncture increases the secretion of nocturnal melatonin, which is a chemical that aids and induces sleep. The study showed that in less than five weeks, regular acupuncture significantly decreased the presence and effects of insomnia in the test study group.

Minimizes Heartburn and Indigestion

Regular acupuncture therapy has been proven to reduce signs of heartburn, indigestion, and required sufferers to use fewer antacids, a recent study shows. Brazilian researchers carried out the test subject and found significant difference between symptoms of pregnant women who used acupuncture, and those who simply watched their diet and took medication when necessary. Although the study was done on pregnant women, the effects are being extrapolated and tested on other test subject groups currently.

Benefits of Acupuncture for Workplace Stress and Pain

Acupuncture can increase your chances of workplace success and offers many benefits to boost your productivity. Acupuncture may also reduce the physical and emotional impacts of an unhealthy or stressful work environment.

1. Reduced Back Pain, Neck Tension and Relieve Joint Pain in the Hands and Arms: Keyboards, heavy backpacks, cell phones, and poor posture are just a few of the culprits that

create the type of pain that penetrates into our workday and keeps us up at night. Acupuncture provides drug-free pain relief while also reduces swelling and inflammation.

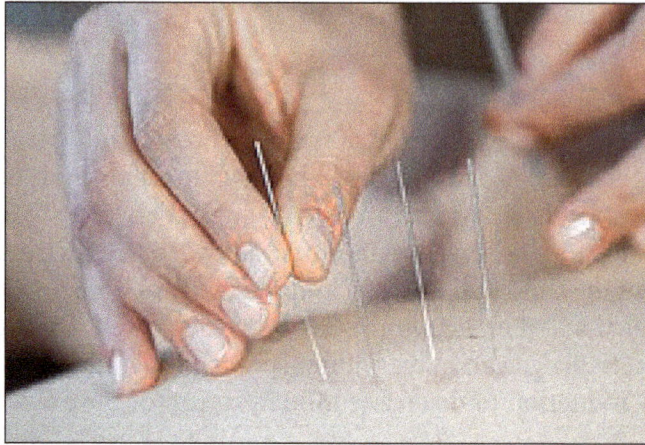

Acupuncture needles are hair-thin and flexible, which means you hardly feel them when inserted.

2. Relief from Headaches: Acupuncture has been used to treat headaches for thousands of years. Recent studies have shown that acupuncture can reduce days with migraines and may have lasting effects. With the most common side effects being a sense of euphoria and relaxation, acupuncture is a choice treatment for those seeking a less invasive, drug-free option.

3. Reduced Eye Strain: Acupuncture can relive eye strain that is often connected to neck tension. Acupuncture also treats many eye ailments including myopia (short-sightedness), hypermetropia (long sightedness), cataract, glaucoma, presbyopia, astigmatism, amblyopia (lazy eye), diplopia, color blindness, and night blindness.

4. Improved Immune System and Reduced Sick Days: Acupuncture can help fight off pathogens by boosting the body's immune system. Acupuncture treatment can also reduce the duration of a cold and relieve debilitating symptoms that keep you feeling miserable and away from work.

5. Enhanced Mental Clarity and Increased Energy: Acupuncture patients report enhanced mental clarity and often experience a surge of increased energy. Improved sleep is additional benefit, which is why acupuncture is used to treat sleep disorders like insomnia.

6. Relief from Digestive Conditions: The link between digestive health and overall health is inescapable. Acupuncture can effectively regulate the digestive system, which is good news for those plagued by gastrointestinal problems.

7. Allergy Relief: Acupuncture can be key in preventing allergies but it is important to being treatments to strengthen your body before allergy season begins. Acupuncture

may also reduce allergy symptoms and can be used in place of or in conjunction with antihistamines.

8. Reduced Cigarette Craving: Acupuncture can be effective in the road to quitting or reducing smoking habits. In addition to helping ease jitters, curb cravings, and lessen irritability, it also promotes lung tissue repair while increasing relaxation and detoxification in the body.

9. Fewer Injuries on the Body Due to Repetitive Strain: Repetitive stress injuries are some of the most common job-related injuries and can lead to a high number of days away from work. Acupuncture is effective in treating repetitive stress injuries and can eliminate the need for surgery or drugs.

Moxibustion

Moxibustion is a kind of external treatment; it is based on the theory of traditional Chinese medicine (TCM), and it usually bakes acupoints with burning moxa wool. Moxibustion can dredge meridians and regulate qi-blood and has been used to prevent and cure diseases for more than 2500 years. Zuo zhuan of the pre-Qin dynasty in China, which recorded a disease discussion occurred in 581 B.C., is considered to be the earliest literature of moxibustion. The silk books discovered in Mawangdui tomb of the Han dynasty (about 168 B.C.), Moxibustion Classic of Eleven Foot-hand Meridians and Prescriptions for Fifty-two Diseases, had documented the use of moxibustion to treat complex diseases. There are a lot of moxibustion contents in Inner Canon of Huangdi; it inferred that the origin of moxibustion is related to the living habits and disease characteristics of northern Alpine nation in the part of Su wen, Yi fa fang yi lun. Later doctors after Han dynasty had made considerable progress in theory and practice on moxibustion and promoted moxibustion to be a mature and widely used therapy.

Moxibustion has been applied in treating a great range of diseases. A bibliometric analysis on the papers published from 1954 to 2007 in China showed that up to 364 kinds of diseases can be treated with moxibustion. The most proper indications of moxibustion therapy are malposition, diarrhea, and colitis; the common proper indications are urinary incontinence and dysmenorrhea; the next common proper indications are knee osteoarthritis, temporomandibular joint disturbance syndrome, soft tissue injury, heel pain, asthma, urinary retention, and herpes zoster. Moxibustion can also be used to treat weakness, fatigue, and aging related problems. Moxibustion can be classified as traditional moxibustion, drug moxibustion, and modern moxibustion. Traditional moxibustion therapy is the most commonly used in the ancient and contemporary moxibustion clinics; it is characterized by the use of moxa as burning material and can be divided into direct moxibustion and indirect moxibustion depending on whether moxa is directly in contact with the skin while operating. A moxa cone placed directly on the skin and ignited is called direct moxibustion, while the moxa kept at certain distance from the skin is called indirect moxibustion. The insulating materials of indirect moxibustion can be air, garlic, ginger, aconite, salt, and so forth. Drug moxibustion, also named nature moxibustion, uses irritant drugs (such as cantharis, garlic, and semen sinapis) to coat the surface of acupoints and make local skin flushed and blistered to cure diseases. Modern moxibustions, such as microwave moxibustion, laser moxibustion, and electrothermal moxibustion, are used to simulate traditional moxibustion stimulation factors by physical or chemical methods to achieve therapeutic effects of moxibustion. Usually, narrow sense of moxibustion refers to the traditional moxibustion with moxa.

Traditional Moxibustion Theory

Ling Shu, Guan Neng says that where needle does not work, moxibustion does. TCM theory holds that moxibustion has a dual effect of tonification and purgation. Different from needles and drugs, characteristics of moxibustion in materials and using fire determine that its efficacy is inclined to warming and nourishing. So, moxibustion is often applied in deficiency-cold syndrome, though some excess-heat syndrome can also use it. The roles of moxibustion can be broadly grouped into warm nourishing, warm dredging, and warm melting. Warm nourishing refers to the benefits of warming Yang, tonifying qi, nurturing blood, and relieving depletion; warm dredging refers to the functions of activating blood, dissolving stasis, promoting qi, dredging channels, and relieving pain; warm melting refers to the roles of reducing phlegm, eliminating stagnation, removing wind, dispelling dampness, drawing out poison, and purging heat. Some people believe that warm dredging is the nature of moxibustion and is the key role of moxibustion effects. The functions of moxibustion, expelling cold, promoting the circulation in meridians and collaterals, clearing away heat, detoxification, and so forth, are dependant on the efficacy of moxibustion for circulating qi and blood flow.

In TCM basic theory, moxibustion effects are based on two aspects: the action of the meridian system and the role of moxa and fire.

Meridian System

TCM usually takes "needling" and "moxibustion" collectively, for both of them are similar therapeutics based on the same theory of meridian and acupoint. In other words, the moxibustion therapeutic effect is partly dependant on the body's nonspecific system of meridians.

Moxibustion is closely related to meridians, cutaneous regions, and acupoints. Meridian system consists of channels and collaterals; they are pathways of communicating internal and external, contacting organs, running qi-blood, and regulating the whole body. Ling Shu, Hai Lun says that there are twelve regular channels, the inner ones belong to viscera and the outer ones connect with limbs. TCM believes that a person is as a whole. The organs and limbs communicate and interact through the meridian system, which plays a very important role in physiological functions and pathological processes. The cutaneous regions are the surface part of the twelve regular channels, which are nourished by channel-qi. The cutaneous regions can show the status of qi-blood from meridians and organs, also it can receive treatment stimulation and then make effects. Acupoints are the sites on the body surface, in which the qi of organs and meridians assembled, that act as target points and response points of treatment.

In the moxibustion treatment process, the cutaneous regions and acupoints are the terminals of the meridian system, as the receivers, by which moxibustion stimulations can be transmitted into the body. Through the meridian system, moxibustion can reinforce insufficiency and reduce excessiveness and directly correct the disease state of the human body or activate the meridian system self-healing function and play a therapeutic role. For example, the different acupoints can cure different diseases in moxibustion, and the same acupoints can get similar results regardless of acupuncture or moxibustion; all of these proved that the body meridian and acupoint system play an important role in the treatment of moxibustion.

Moxa and Fire

Elementary Medicine believes that the diseases that cannot be cured by drugs and acupuncture should be treated with moxibustion. The unique therapeutic effects of moxibustion are closely related to the specificity of moxa and fire.

On moxibustion fire in TCM, there is a discussion in Shen jiu jing lun stating that moxibustion using fire, for being hot and rapid, with soft body can bear with that to eliminate the shadow; it can move instead of stay and always go into organs. Fire is hot, so it can warm back the Yang and eliminate cold of the Yin, even it can melt the poisoning things caused by damp, wind, phlegm, and so on; fire is speedy, so it can dredge the channels, remove the pain or numbness, and active blood and qi. So, the feature of moxa fire shows the main role of moxibustion.

Materials are very important to moxibustion. The choosing of materials of moxibustion in TCM is really harsh. Pu ji fang, Acupuncture cited the Xiao pin fang on eight kinds of fire: moxibustion with pine wood fire, hard to cure; cedar wood fire, ulcer and pus; orange wood fire, skin hurt; mulberry wood, muscle withered; jujube wood fire, body emaciated; bamboo fire, tendons injured, excessive lead tendons flabby; trifoliate orange wood fire, veins "collapse"; elm wood fire, bone hurt, excessive lead bone withered; none of them can be used. But moxa fire is warm without dry, and it can ascend and descend with strong penetration ability into the viscera. Compendium of Materia Medica had said that moxa leaf are slightly bitter and over-spicy when raw, and slightly spicy and over-bitter when processed. Moxa with the nature of pure Yang, raw moxa is warm and become hot after processing. It can take the Tai-Yang fire and get back dying Yang. It can go through three Yin, get rid of all the cold and dampness, and turn the cold into warm after taking orally. Moxibustion with moxa leaf can get into the channels and cure hundreds of diseases. Its function is great. The drug properties of moxa leaves (raw) are that they turn warmer after being processed, become moxa wool (processed), which are suitable for moxibustion, and the older the better. The ancients chose moxa as moxibustion material for it is easy to collect and more for its drug properties, and long-term clinical practices have proved that.

Mechanism Research of Moxibustion

Modern research of moxibustion started in the earlies of last century, Japanese scholars began to observe physical characteristics of moxibustion materials and the effects of moxibustion on blood pressure and intestinal peristalsis in 1912. Up to this day, there have been more and more studies of effects of moxibustion on the human body or experimental animals, almost involving all major physiological systems, especially in the fields of analgesic, enhancing immunity and antiaging. At the same time, researching works on the mechanism of moxibustion also gradually developed, mainly related to the thermal effects, radiation effects, and pharmacological actions of moxa and its combustion products.

Thermal Effects

Burning moxa without flame can produce high temperature of about 548–890°C; it will give a warm feeling when it isclose to the body, so some people think that this treatment is essentially a thermal physical effect. Experiment confirmed that single Zhuang (a dose unit of moxibustion) of moxa cone (2 mg) moxibustion on mice abdomen can raise the temperature to 130°C outside the skin of the point and 56°C inside the skin; the same changes of temperature were not observed in the forelimb far away from the stimulation site. By using 50 mg moxa cone direct moxibustion on the skin of mice with thermocouple implanted, the temperatures of epidermal, subcutaneous, and basal layers were different; the results suggested that moxibustion thermal stimulation affects both shallow and deep tissues of the skin. The maximum temperature change by indirect moxibustion was about 65°C on the skin and 45°C in the subcutaneous layer. The temperature-time curve of moxa cone can be characterized by slow rising, rapid rising, rapid decline, and slow decline phases, and ginger-separated moxibustion can "buffer" the temperature changes. The actual temperature of indirect moxibustion is greatly affected by the texture, size, and the moisture content of the insulating material.

The thermal effects of different moxibustions are not the same. Some people used thermal resistor thermometer and computer online real-time processing to measure the skin temperature at the acupoints of different moxibustions: direct moxibustion, ginger-separated moxibustion, suspension moxibustion, light moxibustion, and He-Ne laser moxibustion. All of them except He-Ne laser moxibustion had significantly changed the temperature of the acupoints through the skin to the muscularis, and each had their own rules and characteristics. The results suggested that the effects on acupoint and even the efficacy of moxibustion depend on the temperature changing of acupoint caused by moxibustion. Others observed the relationship between the moxibustion effect and the intensity of thermal stimulation through the change of pain threshold. In the 40-60 minutes of moxibustion, the pain threshold rose with the operative time and increasing the burning moxa amount per unit time can significantly improve the immediate analgesic effect and lingering effects. Experiment of activation of subnucleus reticularis dorsalis (SRD) neuron by variety intensities of moxibustion thermal stimulation shown that noxious thermal (44–52°C) stimulation can activate SRD neurons, which reaches a plateau when the stimulated area is increased to a certain range.

The warm-heat effect of moxibustion has a close relation to the warm receptors (WRs) and the polymodal receptor (PRs). The antipyretic and thermolytic effects of moxibustion are achieved by stimulating polymodal receptors of acupoints. Effects of moxibustion on the skin can appear as hottness, flushing, pain, blisters, and other skin irritations and burns phenomena. Moxibustion can lead to vasoconstriction at the burning point while vasodilatation around the point and increase peripheral arterial blood flow and microvascular permeability. Another thermal effect of moxibustion is to induce heat shock proteins (HSPs) in local tissues. HSPs are a class of functionally related proteins involved in the folding and unfolding of other proteins. As an endogenous protective mechanism, HSPs can be synthesized in cells in response to hyperthermia and other environmental stresses. The HSPs induced by moxibustion may be an important factor of its mechanism of action.

Radiation Effects

By irradiating acupoints of pain model rats with radiogenic heat of 40–43°C, there are no significant changes in the tail-flick latency or vocalization threshold, suggesting that not any thermal stimulation can achieve moxibustion efficacy. The burning moxa emits visible light and infrared (IR) radiation; therefore, besides the heat effects, nonthermal radiation effect may be an important role in the efficacy of moxibustion. Physics tells us that the radiation is a process of energy outward diffusion in the form of electromagnetic waves or particles; any object above absolute zero in temperature emits electromagnetic radiation. At present, the common view is that the ignited moxa radiation spectrum ranges from 0.8 to 5.6 μm; peak is nearby 1.5 μm, lying within the near infrared (NIR) portion. But results are reported differently due to the measurement methods and the experimental conditions. Thermal radiation of burning moxa stick measured by indirect methods is mainly far infrared (FIR) near NIR, with spectrum peak at 2.8 μm. Measured with visible-infrared monochromator, radiation spectrum of drug moxa sticks is distributed from red light through NIR to middle infrared (MIR), in which multipeaks especially at 2.4 μm are detected and without the parts of wavelength shorter than 0.6 μm.

By analyzing and comparing the infrared radiation spectrums of the moxibustion, the substitute moxibustion, and acupoints of human body, it was found that there was a surprising consistency in the spectrums of three types of indirect moxibustion, namely, separated with prepared monkshood, ginger, and garlic, and the unified spectrum of acupoints. Both had their peaks of radiation near 7.5 μm (after modification, this wavelength should be around 10 μm). However, the spectrum of the substitute moxibustion (separated with cucumber and carrot) was completely different from them. Its warming function was far less than the traditional moxibustion, and there was also a big difference between the infrared radiation spectrums of the moxa-stick (with a peak at 3.5 μm) and acupoints. The results indicated that, in the therapeutic effect of traditional indirect moxibustion, the resonance vibrations of infrared radiation of indirect moxibustion and acupoints play an important role and the substitute moxibustion could not replace the traditional moxibustion in terms of the infrared characteristics of moxibustion.

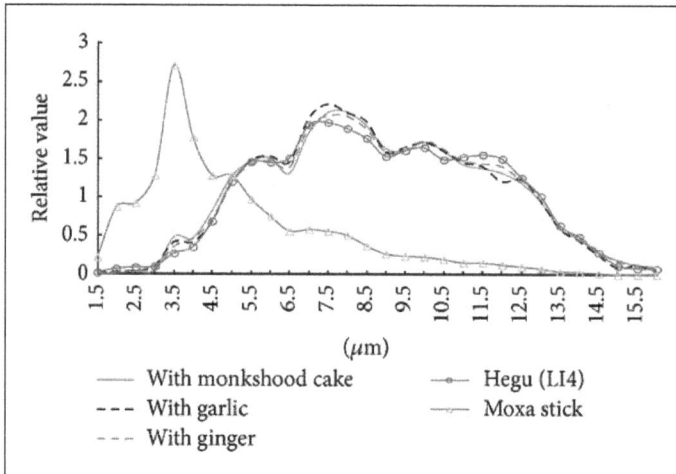

Unified infrared radiation spectrums of an acupuncture point, Hegu (LI 4), direct moxibustion with a traditional moxibustion stick, and indirect moxibustion with three traditional media.

Table: Intensities and peaks wavelengths of the infrared radiation of traditional moxibustion, moxibustion with controls, and Hegu (LI4).

	n	Intensity of radiation (mV)	Wavelength of the peak of radiation (μm)
Traditional moxa stick	4	43300.41 ± 425.15	3.5
Smokeless moxa stick	4	31.15 ± 3.49[#]	7
555 cigarette	4	37.03 ± 3.82[#]	3.5

Indirect moxibustion with monkshood cake	4	681.87 ± 47.52[**ΔΔ]	8
Indirect moxibustion with ginger	4	520.27 ± 68.22[*Δ]	7.5
Indirect moxibustion with garlic	4	594.79 ± 44.71[**ΔΔ]	7.5
Indirect moxibustion with cucumber	4	274.47 ± 19.61	5
Indirect moxibustion with carrot	4	50.53 ± 4.68	5
LI4 (Hegu)	28	20.40 ± 5.69	7.5

#Compared to the traditional moxa-stick, $P = 0.000$.

*Compared to indirect moxibustion with cucumber, $P = 0.004$.

**Compared to indirect moxibustion with cucumber, $P = 0.000$.

ΔCompared to indirect moxibustion with carrot, $P = 0.001$.

ΔΔCompared to indirect moxibustion with carrot, $P = 0.000$.

Infrared acting on the body will produce thermal and nonthermal effects. Thermal effects are produced under the action of electromagnetic waves; the human body molecules absorb energy from IR and convert it into heat and therefore promote blood circulation and improve the cell and enzyme activities. The nonthermal effect is related to the interaction of electromagnetic waves and organism; it is more complex and with nonlinear characteristics. The actions of NIR and FIR on organism are different. NIR is generally believed to play a major role in the biological radiation effect of moxibustion. When NIR irradiates body, the light reflected by the skin is relatively low, the energy can be transmitted about 10 mm deep into the skin, reach the tissues, and be absorbed by them. The NIR can induce some active substances produced within the tissues, after being absorbed by connective tissue, blood vessels, lymphatic vessels, and nerves under the irradiated skin, distribute to other parts of the body with the blood circulation, and enhance the metabolism and thermogenesis of organs they reached. NIR can also energize the metabolism of cells. The energy generated by the photoelectric effect and photochemical process and passed through the nerve-humoral system can provide the activation for the pathological cells lacking energy and then further adjust the body's immune and neurological functions.

Pharmacological Actions

Moxa, *Artemisia argyi* Levl.et Vant., also known as mugwort, is a Compositae *Artemisia* perennial herb. Mugwort leaf can produce moxa wool after drying and grinding, which is a common moxibustion material. The ingredients of moxa are complicated; more than 60 kinds of components had been identified. The volatile oils of moxa include 1,8-Cineole, alkenes (alpha-thujene, pinene, sabinene, etc.), camphor, borneol, and little aldehydes, ketones, phenols, alkanes, and benzene series compounds. Heptatriacontane ($C_{37}H_{76}$) plays an important role in combustion. The moxa also has tannins, flavonoids, sterols, polysaccharides, trace elements, and other ingredients.

The ingredients of moxa always change according to the place and season of production. The oil rate of QiAi in Hubei is obviously higher than in Hebei, Shangdong, and other places. Some people had measured the heat of combustion from different kinds of moxa: QiAi (from Hubei) was 18139 J/g, BeiAi was 17463.4 J/g, QiAi (from Hebei) was 17419.3 J/g, and ChuanAi was 16136.4 J/g. The combustion heat of QiAi (from Hubei) was the biggest, and it has been considered to be the best moxibustion material since ancient times.

The volatile oil rate of moxa is 0.45%–1.00%. It has a variety of biological activities such as the expansion of airway smooth muscle, relieving cough, expectorant effect, and a strong antioxidant activity. The moxa is rich in flavonoids and polysaccharides, which have strong antioxidant activity too.

The moxa combustion test showed that the relative equilibrium moisture content of moxa was 13.51%, the relative ash content was 11.77%, and the relative smoke production rate was 126.42%. Parts of the moxa combustion products are brown tar-like substances; they play a role by penetrating into the human body through the skin damaged by the burning. The moxa and the combustion products of moxa having been extracted with methanol, both extracts showed the actions of clearing the free radicals and lipid peroxidation, and the latter was stronger. The result indicated that the active ingredients of moxa were increased rather than being destroyed after burning. The methanol extracts of moxa combustion products, tars, can be divided with silica gel column chromatography, and the antioxdant components were found in band IV. Further divided by thin-layer chromatography, the antioxidant effect in band Rf 0.14 is better than the synthetic antioxidant BHT. Ginger and garlic, the important auxiliary materials for moxibustion, are commonly used in indirect moxibustion. The ginger and garlic had been put on the evaporating dish for experiment and had confirmed that gingerol and allicin, the active ingredients of them, could act on the body by heat to give the therapeutic effects. The extracts of moxa combustion ashes also have the strong ability of antifree radical.

Another combustion product of moxa is smoke. The smoke of moxa contains a variety of complex components, and its volatile ingredients are ammonia, alcohols (ethylene glycol, pentyl butanol), aliphatic hydrocarbons, aromatic hydrocarbons, terpene compounds and their oxides, and so forth. They may come from the incomplete combustion products of moxa volatile oil of moxa and its oxidation products. Qualitative analysis of the smoke of burning moxa by solid phase microextraction-gas chromatography-mass spectrometry (SPME-GC-MS) had isolated 61 peaks and identified 26 ingredients. The founded substances can be divided into 3 parts by time: The furan structure substances in 0–10 min, mainly aromatic compound in 10–40 min, and esters, alkanes, or hydroxyl-containing compounds in 40–70 min. The smoke of moxa can be used in air disinfection and as antiviral and antifungal. It was also reported that it has applications in wound infections, vaginal itching, uterine prolapse, anal fistula, common warts, and so forth, and some studies showed that the smoke of moxa would make effects on the body through breathing.

There is still a debate on the safety of moxa smoke. Some reports showed that moxa smoke may be harmful to the human body, such as causing allergic reactions. The mugwort leaf contains terpenes; it may produce polycyclic aromatic carcinogens in the process of combustion, and during moxibustion, the concentration of air pollutants, such as nitrogen oxides, carbon monoxide, and particulates, is tenfold higher than the level of standard class II which was issued in the State Environmental Protection Act. They would do damage to the patients and staffs. But a research giving consideration to short-term and long-term exposure showed that the volatile matter and carbon monoxide generated by the smoke of moxa under normal operating conditions did not exceed the safety level.

On the mechanism of moxibustion effects, there have been many viewpoints, such as thermal stimulation effect, non-specific autologous protein therapeutics, non-specific stress responses, and aromatherapy. The generally accepted view is that the meridian system combines with moxibustion physical and chemical effects to produce comprehensive effects. When physical and chemical factors act on the acupoint receptors, the signal enters the central nervous system through the peripheral pathways and outgos after being integrated, adjusting the nerve-endocrine-immune network and circulatory system, so as to regulate the internal environment of the body, in order to achieve the effects of preventing and curing diseases. Although lots of research works have been carried out and made some progress, there is still a great distance from fully understanding the mechanism of moxibustion. Therefore, we will propose the following views on the study of mechanism of moxibustion in the future.

First, value the importance of whole, moxibustion cannot be separated from the theory of TCM. More than a simple stimulus, meridian and acupoint system of the human body is the key of efficacy of moxibustion. The studying of mechanism of moxibustion from the overall level, based on the further understanding of the meridian system or even of the TCM system, is indeed very difficult. But on the other hand, maybe the studies of moxibustion should be helpful to the understanding of acupoint, meridian, and TCM. For example, some people had reported the phenomenon of "heat-sensitive points"; it is a useful exploration of extending the study perspective from the part to the whole with moxibustion as the breakthrough point.

Second, pay more attention to scarring moxibustion (suppurative moxibustion). Scarring moxibustion had been the favorite to ancient doctors, "where there is moxibustion sore, there is cure." Modern clinical practice has also shown that scarring moxibustion, compared with other moxibustions, has advantage of curative effect in the treatment of some chronic refractory diseases.

Third, it is necessary to introduce more new technologies and disciplines into the mechanism research of moxibustion effect, such as bioheat transfer theory, the interdiscipline focus heat transfer phenomena in living organisms; its purpose is to reveal the rules of energy transport in the organisms by introducing the basic theory and research methods of the heat transfer into the field of biology and medicine. The application of the interdisciplinary approach will undoubtedly promote the research of moxibustion.

Fourth, study on the mechanism of moxibustion should be oriented to promote its clinical application. Many research achievements have already been applied in clinic, such as the applications of 650 nm–10.6 μm combined laser moxibustion on knee osteoarthritis and bradycardia and the multifunctional moxibustion instrument which simulate the traditional moxibustion by heating artificial moxa (contains effective components of moxa) with electromagnetic-heating device. There are enough reasons to believe that, with the progress of mechanism research, the new achievements will surely provide a larger space to improve the patient experience and the curative effect of moxibustion.

Health Benefits of Moxibustion

Relieve Pain Instantly

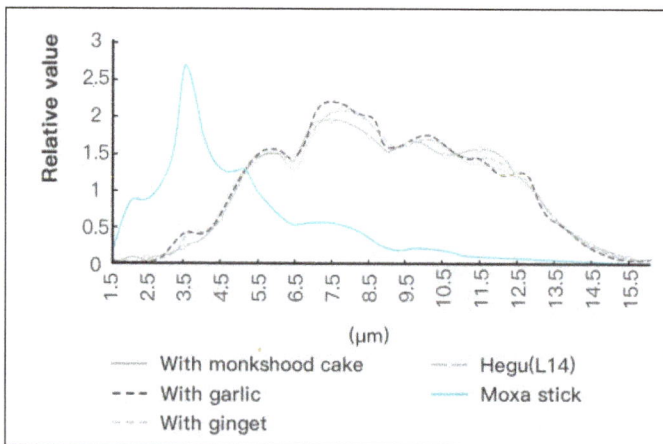

Moxibustion is a form of acupuncture that has been used by therapists and doctors for thousands of years. It improves the flow of Qi, which is the energy in the body, by the heating moxa that causes stimulation in the nerves and releasing endorphins to block pain.

Women's Health: Infertility, Menstrual Cramps, Ovarian Cysts and Breech Births

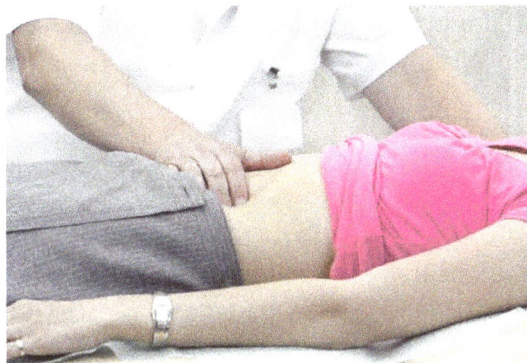

Moxibustion is often touted as a means of decreasing risk of a breech birth. But in a report scientists found insufficient evidence to support the use of moxibustion in correcting a breech presentation. The report's authors sized up three clinical trials (involving a total of 597 women) and concluded that more research is needed before moxibustion can be recommended to women looking to avoid a breech birth. However, the report did find that moxibustion may reduce the need for certain medical procedures typically used to correct a breech presentation.

Improve Immune System

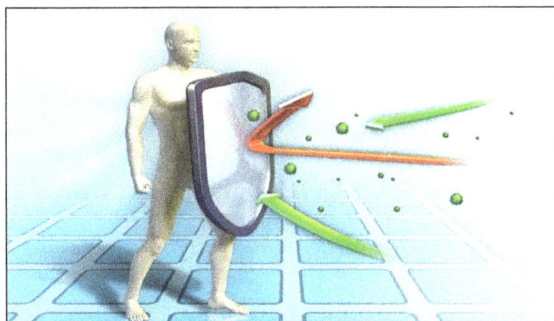

There is a robust history from ancient China and Japan that talks about the daily usage of moxibustion on an acupuncture point called Stomach 36 (Zu San Li). This point is located one hand-width below the patella within the depression on the lateral side of the bone (tibia). This simple daily self-care routine is one of Chinese Medicines' most "famous" preventative therapies.

The daily usage of indirect or direct moxa on this point helps to increase ones vitality and longevity. Some of This points' actions and indications are known to help stimulate the immune system, enhance digestion as well as help treat diarrhea and constipation. It can also increase endurance, alleviate cramps, regulate the bodies Qi, disperse stagnation, and help alleviate pain from the legs and knees.

Accelerate your Recovery and Relax your Mind

The smoldering moxa stick is held over specific areas, often, though not always, corresponding to certain acupuncture points. The glowing end of the moxa stick is held about an inch or two above the surface of the skin until the area reddens and becomes suffused with warmth.

Other Benefits

- Stops the spreading of infection from acute or chronic diseases, and alleviates pain. Also, expels coldness and blood stasis.

- Helps in normalizing or lowering blood pressure.

- Activates and strengthens the body's cells to heal wounds faster.

- Helps in weight loss and weight control.

- Helps increase white and red blood cells to strengthen the hemoglobin and fight against anemia.

- Works as an enhancement for digestive diseases. Helps regulate the stomach and intestine which in return strengthens the digestive system.

- Clears negative blood and toxins from the body.

- Helps treat health conditions related to a weak kidney or high blood pressure.

- Helps weaken cancer cells through the moxa's heat. Studies indicated that applying moxibustion directly on top of the cancer mass will weaken the cancer cells.

- Treats AIDS and Virus diseases. Helps multiple white blood cells.

- Protects the body from contagious diseases.

- Strengthens the body's metabolism and helps in restoring the body's youth.

- Treats alcoholic substance abuse and pesticide addiction by releasing toxins from the body.

- Treats various skin-related conditions: acne, aging spots, wrinkles.

- Increases growth hormones in the body.

- Changes and normalizes acidic blood to alkali blood.

- Improves heart diseases by producing more adrenalin and expanding the blood vessel.

- Expands the capillary vessel and helps the blood stream to travel freely.

References

- What-is-acupuncture: takingcharge.csh.umn.edu, Retrieved 30 April, 2019

- What-types-pain-does-acupuncture-help, treatments, patient: practicalpainmanagement.com, Retrieved 14 July, 2019

- Earacu, tcmbasics, education: acupuncture.com, Retrieved 11 January, 2019

- The-benefits-of-ear-acupuncture: verywellhealth.com, Retrieved 18 April, 2019

- Electroacupuncture takeaway, health: healthline.com, Retrieved 7 May, 2019

- Long-term-benefits-acupuncture: independentfemme.com, Retrieved 21 July, 2019

- Acupuncture: organicfacts.net, Retrieved 13 July, 2019

- Top-10-benefits-acupuncture-workplace-stress-pain: alignedmodernhealth.com, Retrieved 24 March , 2019

- Benefits-of-moxibustion, news: ijoou.store, Retrieved 13 June, 2019

Chapter 5

Diagnosis in Traditional Chinese Medicine

The diagnosis in traditional Chinese medicine makes use of numerous diagnostic methods, such as the examination of the tongue and the pulse. This chapter closely examines the key concepts related to these diagnostic methods in traditional Chinese medicine as well as the eight principles of diagnosis to provide an extensive understanding of the subject.

Causes of Disease in Chinese Medicine

In Traditional Chinese Medicine (TCM), this "lottery theory" has credence; Ancestral Qi, or DNA, influences your probability of falling victim to disease. At the same time, you could have great Ancestral Qi and make poor lifestyle choices that create disease. Even if you have a familial disposition to disease, you can choose to practice Qi Gong exercises, eat whole foods, and using tonic herbs as preventative and corrective strategies to create healthy aging and good health throughout your life.

Chinese medicine is a complex system that relies on many methods to keep the body in "balance". If the body is in harmony or balance, it is able to resist pathogens (agents that produce disease) and will not develop chronic diseases that will lead to premature aging and degeneration. Wellness in Chinese medicine does not simply refer to an absence of disease; rather, a healthy person is happy, healthy and pain-free. There is an understanding in Chinese medicine that wellness is a natural state and illness is the result of any number of influences. In an effort to understanding how to obtain wellness, we will explore how a person can develop diseases and imbalances.

Emotions Causing Disease according to Chinese Medicine

In Chinese medical theory, one of the major internal causes of disease is the Seven Emotions: anger, worry, fear, fright, anxiety, grief, and joy. All of these emotions are normal and everyone experiences them at different times. They can only cause disease and injure the vital organs if the emotional responses are out of normal proportion or deficient in response to the situation, or they are chronic in nature. Likewise, if an organ system becomes deficient or out of balance, the related emotions can occur chronically; it is often the "chicken or the egg" dilemma trying to determine if a bodily imbalance caused abnormal emotional response, or if the emotions damaged the organ system. All of the emotions originate in the Heart, and serious emotional disorders are considered "Heart Shen" disorders.

Anger

If someone walks up to you and slaps you in the face, you would likely be angry for a few hours and then move on with your life. If you do not become angry when attacked by another, that could show an imbalance. If you carry anger around for weeks, or even worse, years, that anger will begin to affect the Liver Function and the physical health of the Liver. Liver imbalances can include other emotional traits in addition to anger such as short temper, frustration, lack of vision, inability to plan and strategies, feeling stuck, depression, inflexibility, or lack of courage.

Worry

It is normal to worry from time to time if the children are out late, or the husband is trying out the new grill, or your plane ride runs into turbulence. However, when worry turns to obsessing and your mind won't turn away from the question, "but what if", then worry could damage the Spleen Function of the body. Likewise, Spleen Deficiency can lead to excessive worry. In Chinese medicine the Spleen is much more complex than western medicine; it is in charge of the transportation of foods and fluids and works closely with the Stomach in its digestive capacity. Worry is also implied with any over thinking or very heavy study patterns that can also damage the Spleen over time. Other emotional traits that are associated with Spleen imbalances would include inability to be empathetic, inability to nurture other, eating disorders, obesity, or not feeling grounded.

Fear, Fright and Anxiety

Fear and anxiety are produced by your own thoughts and the mind's ability to speculate on possible negative outcomes of a situation. Fright is produced by a shock, such as a dog trying attacking you, or extreme sport opportunities such as skydiving and is normal in those circumstances. Prolonged exposure to fear will damage the Kidney System in Chinese medicine. Likewise, Kidney Deficiency and Kidney imbalances can manifest in to anxiety, panic attacks, sexual disorders and lack of willpower. Even the lack of awe, such as the inability to appreciate a beautiful sunset, is a sign that the Kidney System is not functioning to its fullest capacity.

Grief and Sadness

The normal response to loss is grief. When we are unable to pass through all of the stages of grief (denial, anger, bargaining, depression and acceptance), we become energetically stuck. If we are stuck in grief for a long period of time, it will begin to damage the Lung Function. Other traits of Lung imbalances could include sadness, low self-esteem, lack of boundaries, inability to "let go", lack of structure or too much structure, rigid belief systems, or critical judgment of others.

Joy

This reference is about happiness, and our ability to experience joy depends on Heart health. Out of balance joy can manifest as mania, as in manic-depressive disorders. When people are manic, there is allot of harmful heat in the heart and the Heart Function is damaged over time. The Heart is actually the origin of all of the emotions and has to be addressed any time there is an emotional disorder. Other signs of Heart Function disorders could include a lack of emotional warmth, a lack of sexual desire or excessive sexual desire, insomnia, sleep disorders and hatred.

External Causes of Disease in Traditional Chinese Medicine

In Traditional Chinese Medicine, everything in the universe is interconnected. Therefore, changes in the universe, such as weather, influence humans. Weather is characterized by six external energies that can cause disharmony in the body. They are known as the Six Pathogenic Factors. These pathogenic factors are opportunistic and can only cause disease when our immune systems are weakened:

- Wind causes symptoms that wander and change.

- Cold causes sudden onset of symptoms of chilliness, headache, and body aches.

- Damp causes sluggishness, lethargy, sticky discharges.

- Heat and Fire symptoms include fever, inflammation, constipation, and dry skin.

- Summer Heat (heat stroke) depletes Qi and Body Fluids, which can cause dehydration and exhaustion.

- Dryness is closely related to Heat but involves more drying of bodily fluids. Symptoms include dry eyes, dry nose, dry mouth, and dry cough.

- Toxins are a more recent addition to the list of six external causes of disease. Toxins are virulent pathogens that are not associated with climactic factors and can attack even the normally resistant individual.

Other Major Causes of Disease in TCM

Genetic Factors

Chinese medicine has recognized the influence of familial disease patterns for thousands of years and practitioners have inquired about family history long before DNA was discovered. Some people are under the false perception that genetic imbalances cannot be positively influenced. Just as a change in diet and exercise can improve the prognosis of the offspring of a heart attack patient, Chinese tonic herbs and other medical techniques can improve the prognosis for all types of genetically related diseases.

Diet

Improper eating habits can cause imbalances in many organ systems. Good eating habits are generally well understood in our culture with recent interest in wellness being a popular topic in the media. Organic, whole foods are always a good idea. Chinese medicine would advise against any excesses such as too much salt which would damage the Kidney function or too many spicy foods that may damage the lungs. Also, iced drinks, excessive raw foods and juices can cause dampness and damage the Spleen function.

Exercise

Proper exercise is important in keeping Blood and Qi flowing. Brisk walking, qigong, tai qi and yoga are the preferred types of exercise in Chinese medicine. Vigorous exercise or very hard physical work can cause imbalances and should be avoided.

Sex

The lack of sexual desire would indicate an imbalance of the Heart Function and Kidney Function. Too much sexual activity can drain the Kidney energy especially for men. Childbirth can be draining for women's Kidney energy.

Sleep

Having sound sleep during the night is a vital part of maintaining wellness in Chinese medicine. Broken sleep patterns, wakefulness at night, or lack of sleep are all reason for concern.

Miscellaneous Causes of Disease

These include trauma, stress, environmental pollutants, parasites, poor posture, drug and alcohol use, and other poor lifestyle habits.

Cold in Traditional Chinese Medicine

The cold pathogenic factor is considered a yin evil qi. Its nature is to slow movement down, causing tightness, contraction, stagnation, and impaired circulation. When it is an external pathogenic factor, cold can attack the skin, muscles, and lungs. When it is an internal pathogenic factor, cold can cause an impairment in the normal functions of the spleen, stomach, and kidneys.

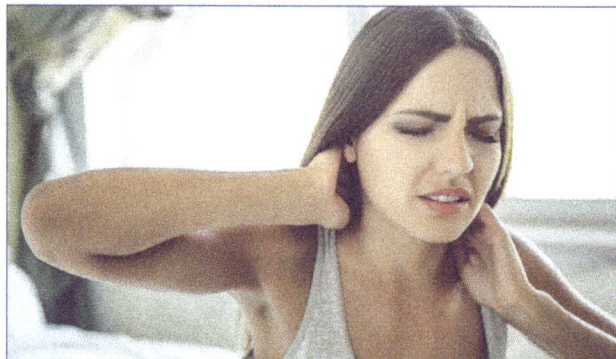

Wind cold can cause tight shoulders and neck.

Syndromes of Cold

1. Wind Cold: In combination with the pathogenic factor of wind, cold attacks the exterior of the body and the lungs, causing chills, lack of sweating, occipital headache (pain at the base of the skull), upper body aches, tight shoulders and neck, and a congested nose. The influence of wind causes the symptoms to appear suddenly and affect the upper body, while cold causes the muscles to contract, causing the stiffness and pain. Nasal secretions are clear - another sign of cold. The treatment principle is to repel the wind and disperse the cold with warm diaphoretic herbs, acupuncture, and moxibustion.

2. Obstruction Due to Cold: Traditionally known as cold bi (blockage) pain, this condition typically takes the form of body aches or joint pain that is relieved by warmth. The most common Western diagnosis for this pattern is arthritis. Since the syndrome is caused by cold, the joint may actually feel cold to the touch, and the pain typically gets worse in cold weather. The Chinese treatment principle is to increase circulation and warm the acupuncture meridians through which qi and blood circulate by means of moxibustion, acupuncture, and herbs.

3. Cold Attacking the Spleen and Stomach: In this externally caused disorder, cold causes digestive symptoms such as abdominal pain, clear vomit, and watery diarrhea. Although it usually accompanies an externally contracted cold or stomach bacteria or virus (what we commonly refer to as stomach "flu"), this syndrome can also be caused by eating cold foods such as ice cream.

4. Cold Congealing the Liver Meridian: The liver meridian passes through the genital area, and this condition is a manifestation of cold in that meridian. Symptoms include testicular pain or shrinking and hernia pain. Moxibustion, acupuncture, and herbs can effectively correct this imbalance in a short time.

5. Spleen Yang Deficiency: If a person has an underlying deficiency of spleen yang (deficiency in energy and heat needed in order to digest food), cold can severely impair digestive function. Symptoms of spleen yang deficiency include watery stools with undigested food,

cold extremities, edema, and a slow pulse. When a person with this underlying deficiency is also affected by external cold pathogens, the imbalance is especially difficult to eliminate.

6. Treatment first expels the cold pathogenic factor. Then it tonifies the yang aspect of the spleen and kidneys to bring about a long-term increase in the body's basic metabolism, or its ability to maintain the heat needed for proper digestion, which is known in traditional Chinese medicine as life-gate (metabolic) fire. Spleen yang deficiency is treated with moxibustion and warming herbs that tonify spleen yang.

7. Kidney Yang Deficiency: Since the kidneys are the source of yang metabolic fire for the entire body, a deficiency in kidney yang can make the individual especially prone to cold. The symptoms of kidney yang deficiency include an inability to stay warm, cold extremities, low sex drive, frequent urination, edema (fluid retention), and pain in the low back. The yang deficiency can be corrected with long-term application of moxibustion and consumption of herbs that tonify kidney yang, thereby increasing metabolic fire.

Poor Dietary Habits

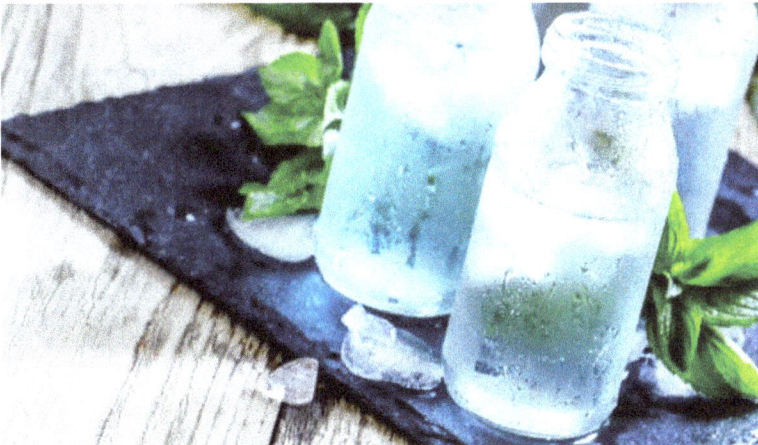

Consumption of cool liquids can disrupt the digestive process.

Poor dietary habits are a major cause of disease. Since food is the medicine we take most often, many illnesses can be quite difficult to treat unless changes occur in a person's diet. Some of the eating and drinking habits that can lead to disease are explained below:

1. Irregular Times and Amounts: It is important to consider the time it takes food to pass through the stomach. Simple fruits and vegetables can leave the stomach after about 20 minutes, while more concentrated proteins, starches, and fats may take 4 to 5 hours. If the stomach contains partially digested food when the person eats another meal, the digestive process can be seriously impaired. This would be similar to getting a small fire started with kindling and then dumping a load of logs on the fire. Even though logs are good fuel, the fledgling fire was not ready for so much fuel.

Conversely, if a person waits too long between meals, secretion of digestive juices stops. This would be akin to letting the kindling go out before putting logs on the fire. We need to eat when the stomach signals true hunger. Consumption of liquids is also an important cause of imbalance. If a person drinks a large glass of cold water after a meal, the digestive juices become diluted. (The stomach secretes just enough enzymes to digest a particular meal.) Also, the stomach needs a certain amount of heat for the chemical reactions of the digestive process to take place; cold liquids slow the reaction. It is best for the contents of the stomach to be a soup-like consistency, since too much dryness can also disturb digestion.

Achieving this consistency can be accomplished by sipping liquids, preferably warm, along with a meal. In China and other Asian countries, it is common to serve soup with almost every meal. If a person desires cool water, the water should be consumed at least half an hour before a meal or three hours after a meal, when the stomach is empty.

2. Consuming the Wrong Types of Food: Foods have different energetic qualities; something appropriate for one type of person or climate might be unhealthy for another body type or weather pattern. For example, cold and raw foods are very healthy in hot weather or for a person who has too much internal heat. Conversely, these foods can deplete the spleen qi and yang and cause dampness in cold weather or in persons who have too much internal cold. In coastal California, for example, residents experience all four seasons in a twenty-four hour day. It might be foggy and cold in the morning, making a breakfast of hot grains or soup an appropriate choice. By midday, it can be sunny and hot, a good time to consume fruits and salads.

Similarly, spicy food is appropriate for cold weather or persons who are yang deficient, but it can cause imbalance in hot weather, especially in persons who have internal heat. This goes to show that no food is always healthy; it is a matter of choosing foods that match the internal and external climates. Certain foods, such as sweets or alcohol, are meant to be used infrequently and in small quantities; overconsumption can cause a wide range of problems.

3. Overeating or Undereating: Malnutrition due to undereating can lead to a chronic deficiency of qi and blood. While more common in developing countries, this condition is also seen in developed countries in conditions of poverty and in persons who suffer from emotional imbalances and substance abuse. Treatment includes herbs that tonify qi and blood, along with an improvement in nutritional intake. In the West, overconsumption is a far more common problem, leading to a high incidence of heart disease, high blood pressure, stroke, diabetes, and cancer. In traditional Chinese medicine, acupuncture is used to reduce cravings; dietary and lifestyle counseling are also important.

4. Food Cravings and Addictions: The human body is designed to process a wide variety of foods to meet our needs. Fad diets or addictions to a narrow range of foods can be

debilitating. Some essential nutrients are likely to be missing from a narrow diet. By eating a wide assortment of different-colored vegetables, whole grains, and proteins, we can receive the nutrition we need to function at a high level of wellness.

5. Contaminated Food: Although more common in developing or tropical countries, parasites are a problem all over the world. They can wreak havoc on the digestive organs, damaging the qi of the spleen and stomach. Herbs that kill parasites are quite strong, so it is important to have an accurate diagnosis through a stool test before beginning treatment. Other sources of contamination are toxins produced by bacterial contamination in the course of processing food. Meats are especially susceptible to this sort of pathogen; you should always cook meat thoroughly to kill virulent microorganisms. Water-borne pathogens are another source of disease, and water of questionable quality should always be boiled.

Treatment of pathogenic microorganisms depends on the type of pathogen involved. In general, gastrointestinal distress caused by microorganisms can be treated with herbal medicines. Although herb formulas can be remarkably effective, they should be considered a first-aid measure until a person can see their health care practitioner.

Lack of Exercise

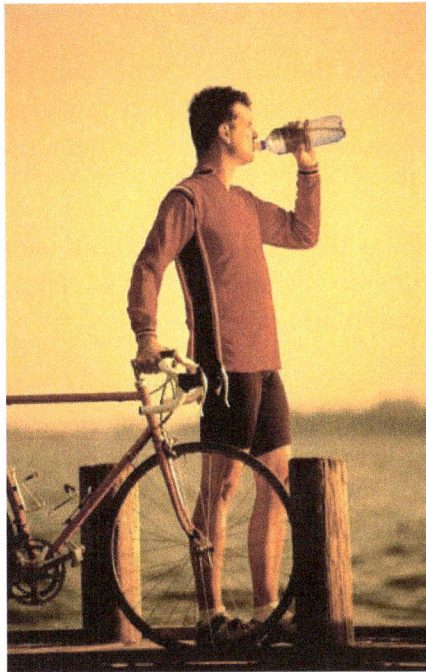

A balanced life, with both exercise and rest, is important for good health.

Too little exercise can lead to stagnation of qi and blood and, subsequently, a variety of degenerative diseases, including obesity, cancer, and heart disease. Moderate exercise strengthens the heart and lungs and stimulates the flow of blood and lymph, the body's filtration system, which filters out toxins. In fact, exercise is the only way to pump lymph through the body, since lymph isn't powered by the heart. Some of the traditional Chinese ideas about lack of exercise are expressed in the ancient texts:

- "Sleeping or lying down too much hurts the qi." When a person oversleeps, he typically feels tired all day.

- "Too much sitting hurts the muscles." This refers to the fact that lack of exercise causes the muscles to atrophy.

- "A running stream doesn't go bad." Stagnant water easily becomes spoiled, and stagnant qi and blood can lead to many different illnesses.

On the other hand, too much activity can hurt the body. This is especially true if a person is fighting a cold or is already depleted and in need of rest. In these cases, almost any exercise can drain the qi. Some of the traditional ideas about excessive activity:

- Using the eyes too much hurts the blood: Since the eyes are intimately connected with the liver, excessive use of the eyes can drain that organ. The liver stores the blood, so stressing it in this way depletes the blood supply.

- Too much standing hurts the bones: People who must stand all day at work, especially on a concrete floor, can vouch for the truth of this statement. Some of the conditions that can be caused by standing too much are sore feet, painful joints, and varicose veins.

- Too much walking hurts the tendons: Tendinitis is a very common condition, especially among runners. Computer work and repetitive stress injuries are also frequent causes of tendon injury.

- Too much work for the heart injures the spirit (shen): Since the heart is the seat of the mind, too much mental work affects the spirit. It is important to get sufficient physical exercise to avoid this imbalance.

- Too much work for the liver hurts the blood: The liver blood can also be depleted by too much work, as can be seen in marathon runners who no longer have menstrual periods. When they ease up on their workouts, their menstrual periods usually return.

- Too much work for the kidneys hurts the essence (jing): Each individual has a different capacity for sexual activity, depending on their age and their constitution. Overindulgence in sexual activity, however, can lead to a depletion of the kidneys, causing fatigue and chronic pain in the low back.

Other Causes of Illness

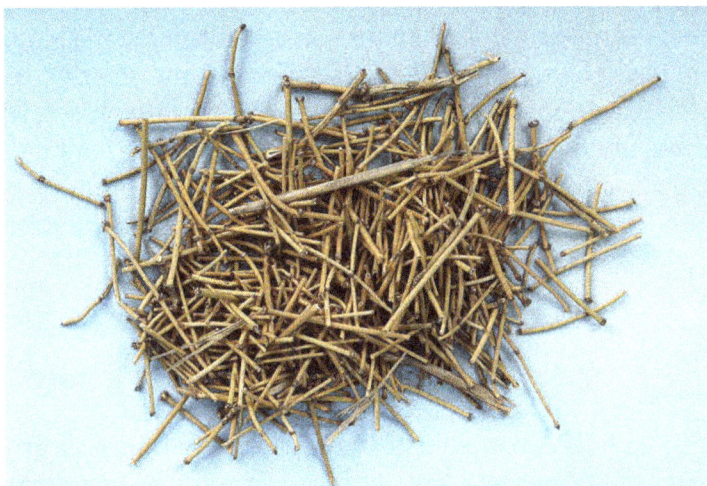

Ephedra is a traditional Chinese medicine herb that can
have both positive and negative side effects.

There are other causes of disease that don't fit within the categories of the six pernicious influences, the seven emotions, exercise, or nutrition.

Predisposition to Disease

We inherit our prenatal qi and essence from our parents. This genetic inheritance is outside our control, and it can be the determining factor in a number of ailments. For example, if a man's grandfather and father both died of heart disease in their 40s, he will be much more likely to develop heart disease than a person with a similar lifestyle whose ancestors lived into their 90s. It is necessary for a person with a weak inherited constitution to pursue a very healthy lifestyle to avoid disease.

Accidents and Injuries

These causes of disease are self-explanatory. However, a person with strong qi and blood will recover from injuries much faster than a person who is deficient in these vital substances. Traditional Chinese medicine is especially effective in treating injuries of all types.

Side Effects of Medical Treatments

This is especially common with Western medicine, where the list of possible side effects for a drug might fill two pages of text. A recent study found that in some hospitals, as many as 30 percent of patients at any given time are receiving treatment for the side effects of the drugs they're taking. Herbal medicine can be very helpful in reducing many of these side effects; cancer patients in Chinese hospitals, for example, are routinely prescribed herbs to help counteract the side effects of chemotherapy.

Although herbal medicine is exceptionally safe, side effects can occur, although they are rarely serious. For example, many herbs are hard to digest and can cause loose stools. An herbalist takes this into account when preparing a formula for a patient, adding specific herbs to counteract these side effects. If herbs are improperly prescribed, on the other hand,the side effects can be more severe. For example, a person who suffers from high blood pressure should never be given the herb Ephedra (ma huang), since it can cause a rise in blood pressure. For this reason, traditional Chinese medical texts also list formulas that are used to counteract the effects of improper treatments.

Diagnosis

Diagnosis in traditional Chinese medicine may appear to be simply a grouping of symptoms, but the elegance of Chinese medicine is that a diagnosis automatically indicates a treatment strategy.

For example, a woman experiencing menopause may have hot flashes, night sweats, thirst, and irritability; this group of symptoms leads to a diagnosis of kidney yin deficiency with heat. This diagnosis immediately points to the indicated therapy: Tonify kidney yin and clear deficiency heat. Since standard formulas are available for this pattern, such as Rehmannia Teapills, an accurate diagnosis enables a practitioner to prescribe a treatment that has been proved safe and effective for thousands of years.

A practitioner can obtain all of the information needed to diagnose disease through inquiry and external observation. The four basic categories of diagnostic observation are looking, listening and smelling, asking, and touching. Simply by employing these four areas of investigation, traditional practitioners can accurately assess physical and emotional imbalances of the internal organs and reestablish harmony.

It is important to remember that diagnostic indicators are always viewed holistically - that is, in total and in relation to the whole person. For example, fatigue is a symptom of qi or blood deficiency, but fatigue is also a symptom in a case of wind cold. If a person with wind-cold was mistakenly diagnosed with qi deficiency, he might be given ginseng, a strong tonic that would make the symptoms much worse.

A careful practitioner would note that the person's pulse was strong and floating, a sign of wind cold, while a person with qi deficiency would have a deep and weak pulse. While it is necessary to learn the individual diagnostic patterns, it is crucial to remember that any sign or symptom must be viewed in relation to the whole person.

Use of Sight in Traditional Chinese Medicine Diagnosis

The use of sight in traditional Chinese medicine diagnosis is crucial. By examining the face, the body, and the tongue, a practitioner can recognize signs and symptoms that indicate illness. Treatment cannot begin until observation using sight has been made and other methods of diagnosis have been employed.

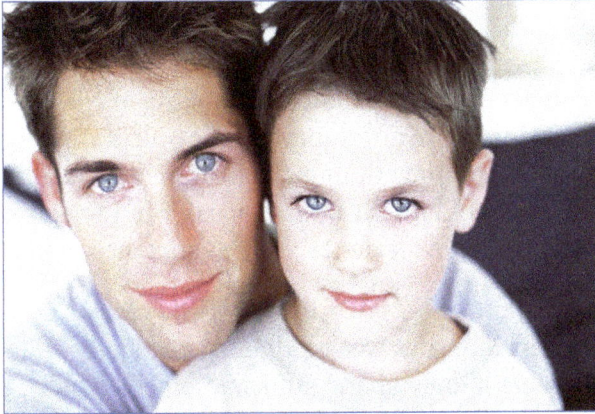

The pallor of the face is just one indicator of a person's overall health.

Face

An experienced practitioner often develops an initial idea of a patient's health just by observing him or her walking into the office. Inspecting the quality of the spirit (shen) is an important aspect of this first impression, since the shen gives a good indication of the overall vitality of a person. The shen especially shows in the eyes: An ancient maxim states, "If there is shen, there is life." A person with healthy shen has a gleam or sparkle of life in the eyes.

The face is bright with some color, breathing is regular, and movements and speech are normal and logical. A person with unhealthy spirit has dim eyes with a vacant look. The face is dull with no shine; breathing is slow, weak, or irregular; movements appear abnormal or unusual; and speech is illogical or the voice is at an inappropriate volume.

Changes in facial skin color can provide the traditional Chinese medicine practitioner with a number of diagnostic clues. A bright (shiny), white face can indicate deficiency of qi or a cold condition, while a dull, pale face with no shine is a sign of blood deficiency.

Redness in the face indicates heat: If the entire face is red, it is a sign of excess heat, while red cheeks alone are a sign of deficiency heat. A bright yellow skin tone can indicate damp heat, while pale yellow is a sign of damp cold due to deficiency. Finally, areas of black usually indicate kidney deficiency.

The location of color on the face also has diagnostic significance as in the example of kidney deficiency. The black appears below the eyes and is often seen in people who don't get enough sleep or push themselves too hard, both practices that deplete the kidneys of qi, yin, and yang. Another example of the importance of the location of color is when it appears on the tip of the nose, an area affected by the spleen. Alcoholics often have redness in this area due to damp heat in the spleen caused by the heat generated in that organ by alcohol.

Body

A lot of information can also be accumulated by looking at the overall physique. Overweight people have a tendency toward dampness or phlegm, while thin people are inclined to be yin deficient. A person with internal heat may be scantily clad in the winter, while a person with internal cold might wear a sweater in the summer. Somebody who is active and energetic tends to experience yang syndromes, while yin syndromes are more common in quiet, sedentary people.

Faded, sparse, and dry hair indicates weak kidney qi or blood, while lustrous, thick, and shiny hair is a sign of strong kidney qi and sufficient blood. Finally, the lips can tell a lot about the condition of the body. Bright red lips can indicate heat, pale lips can be a sign of qi or blood deficiency, and blue lips can be due to cold or blood stagnation. Dry and cracked lips are a sign of depleted body fluids, and twitching lips are an indication of liver wind.

Use of Sound and Smell in Traditional Chinese Medicine Diagnosis

The use of sound and smell in traditional Chinese medicine can garner information when diagnosing a patient. The two diagnostic tools are grouped together because the same Chinese word is used for both of them. In this diagnostic area, the practitioner listens to the various sounds emanating from the patient and pays attention to any unusual smells. A wealth of information can be gleaned from these perceptions, and they give the physician some clues to pursue later on during the initial interview.

Speaking

A person under attack by an external pathogen speaks softly at first, with the voice gradually becoming louder. With an internal deficiency, the voice gets softer over time due to a lack of energy. People with cold syndromes tend to be quiet, while heat syndromes are associated with excessive talking. It is the nature of cold to slow functions and movement, while heat speeds them up.

A person with an excess condition tends to have a loud, strong voice, while a soft, weak voice is associated with deficiency patterns. Repeated sighing is often a sign of liver qi stagnation; it is an attempt by the body to release pent-up emotion while expanding the chest muscles that tighten due to the stagnation.

Breathing: Weak and shallow breathing that is difficult to hear is associated with deficiency, especially of the lungs and kidneys. Loud and heavy breathing indicates an excess condition that constricts the air passages. The source of asthmatic wheezing can also be differentiated by its sounds. In a deficiency pattern, the sound is soft and the patient experiences difficulty inhaling due to the kidneys' inability to "grasp the qi."

In a lung excess syndrome, the wheezing is coarse and loud and the patient has difficulty exhaling. A loud cough is a sign of excess, while a weak, slow cough is due to deficiency. A dry, hacking sound can indicate dryness or yin deficiency, while gurgling sounds are a sign of phlegm.

Gastrointestinal Signs: Vomiting due to an excess condition is loud and strong, while a deficiency condition causes vomiting that is weak and painful. Hiccups are known as "rebellious stomach qi" in traditional Chinese diagnosis. If they are due to excess, the sound is loud and short, while deficiency hiccups have a weak sound and last longer. If hiccups show up in an illness after a few days, it is an indication of a collapse of stomach qi. Loud belching is a sign of excess; if there is heat, a sour smell accompanies the belching. Deficiency belching has a softer sound with no sour smell.

Smelling

In general, strong smells are due to heat, while a lack of aroma is a sign of cold. This applies to the breath, urine, stools, vomit, sweat, and any discharges. Some specific smells are linked to organs; for example, a sweet smell is linked to the spleen, a urine-like smell is associated with a kidney problem, and a smell like rotten apples is a sign of diabetes ("wasting and thirsting syndrome").

Asking

This is an exceptionally important aspect of diagnosis, for Western as well as traditional Chinese practitioners. When interviewing the patient, the traditional Chinese practitioner accumulates enough information to formulate a diagnosis based on the condition of the internal organs, pernicious influences, and vital substances.

The traditional Chinese practitioner also delves further into information that he or she uncovered while "looking, listening, and smelling." In addition, the practitioner attempts to get an accurate picture of the person's past medical history, lifestyle, and present area of complaint, gradually building a complete diagnostic picture.

Use of Physical Factors in Traditional Chinese Medicine Diagnosis

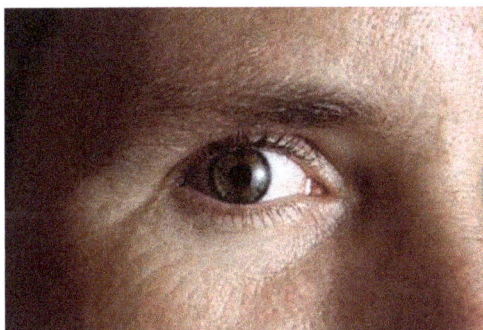

The eyes aren't just the window to the soul. They tell a practitioner if you're sick or not.

Evaluating physical factors in traditional Chinese medicine is important to making a diagnosis. These factors can indicate the type and level of an illness.

Chills and Fever

It is important to remember that these terms refer more to the patient's perceptions of cold or heat, rather than an actual elevated body temperature or shivering. Chills and fever that occur simultaneously indicate an external condition. If the chills are worse than the fever, the condition is wind cold; if the fever is worse than the chills, it is wind heat.

In either case, if the fever persists after the chills disappear, it is a sign that the condition has penetrated to the interior of the body. If the fever persists and is accompanied by sweating, thirst, and constipation, the interior heat has penetrated to the stomach and intestines, which is an even deeper level.

A chronic low-grade fever can occur after an illness accompanied by a fever has "burned out the yin." This sort of fever can also be a sign of qi deficiency associated with a collapse of the body's immune system. Feeling cold can be a symptom of either wind cold or yang deficiency. In wind cold, it can be difficult for a person to get warm, even when he or she is bundled up in warm clothes. Wind cold is an acute ailment of short duration, while yang deficiency is a long-term, chronic condition.

Perspiration

Perspiration is regulated through the opening and closing of the pores, a function of the defensive qi (wei qi). When qi or yang deficiency occurs, the pores remain open due to weakness, and the person experiences spontaneous sweating during the day. This can occur even if the person has not become overheated. Sensations of heat in the evening with night sweats are considered a sign of yin deficiency. This condition is called "stealing sweats" because it steals fluids from the body like a thief in the night.

In an external disorder, perspiration is an important indicator of the final diagnosis: With wind heat, the person perspires, while with wind cold, the pores are closed from cold, causing a lack of sweating. If sweating occurs with an external condition, and the person feels better afterward, it is a sign that the body has successfully expelled the pathogen. If sweating doesn't break the fever or make the person feel better, the pathogen is successfully fighting against the wei qi.

Head and Body

Headaches that have an acute onset with severe pain are usually due to an external pernicious influence, such as wind cold or wind heat. Milder, more chronic headache pain suggests an internal influence such as qi or blood deficiency. Severe, intermittent pain is likely due to liver fire, which rises up to the head, often from an outburst of anger.

The location of the headache also has clinical significance, since it helps the physician select herbs and acupuncture meridians that run through the area of pain. For example, a frontal headache is considered a disorder of the stomach meridian. Treatment involves needling acupuncture points on that meridian and prescribing herbs with an affinity for that area of the body. Pain at the top or sides of the head is related to the liver and gallbladder, while pain at the back of the head is related to the bladder meridian.

Dizziness is another important diagnostic aspect associated with the head. If dizziness is due to qi deficiency, the symptoms are mild and get worse when the person is tired. Blood deficiency dizziness is also mild and gets worse when the person stands up suddenly. Dizziness from dampness is associated with a heavy feeling, which patients often describe as a "wet blanket wrapped around the head." Liver fire can create a severe form of dizziness in which the person loses balance as if on a rolling ship. If the head itself is shaking, it is a sign of internal wind moving.

Since many people turn to traditional Chinese medicine for the treatment of pain, this is often the first symptom mentioned to a practitioner. The practitioner can accumulate an abundance of information by asking about the location, severity, frequency, and causes of pain in the patient's body. Pain that comes and goes is due to wind or qi stagnation, while pain in a fixed location is a result of cold or blood stagnation. If pressure relieves the pain, it is a deficient type; pressure always makes excess type pain feel worse. Pain in specific areas of the body can also serve as a sign of problems in an internal organ.

For example, pain in the rib area is a symptom of stagnation in the liver and gallbladder. Lower back pain is a cardinal sign of kidney deficiency. Since it is due to depletion, it gets worse after exertion. When low back pain is due to cold and dampness, a stagnant condition, it gets worse after rest.

Ears and Eyes

Since the kidneys open up into the ears, poor hearing or deafness is usually from kidney deficiency. Sudden deafness is usually due to heat and fire rising up to the ears, which is an excess condition. Similarly, ringing in the ears (tinnitus) is a sign of an excess condition if it comes on suddenly as a loud, high sound. Most often this is a condition of liver yang rising up to the head. Development of tinnitus over a long time is a sign of depletion of the kidneys. One diagnostic test is to press on the ears. If the sound gets stronger, it is due to excess; if it gets weaker, it is due to deficiency.

The eyes can also tell a lot about the patient. As previously mentioned, a practitioner looks into the eyes to assess the state of a person's shen (spirit) and thus acquire a general picture of the overall vitality and the potential for healing. Pain in the eyes can be due to liver fire or wind heat, while dry eyes can be caused by blood deficiency. Poor vision in general is associated with kidney jing or liver blood deficiency, as is night blindness. Itching in the eyes is a symptom of external wind or blood deficiency. Abnormal eye movement is a sign of internal wind.

Stools and Urine

The stools and urine are important sources of information but may be signs overlooked by the patient. Stools that are sticky or cause burning with a strong smell are a sign of heat, while watery diarrhea with little smell is a sign of deficiency or cold. Damp heat causes frequent urges to defecate, but only a small amount is expelled each time. Stools that are watery with undigested food indicate spleen yang deficiency; if the same symptoms occur early in the morning ("cock's crow diarrhea"), it is due to kidney yang deficiency.

When constipation occurs, other diagnostic signs must be taken into account. If constipation accompanies dark urine, bad breath, and a yellow tongue coat, heat is the cause. Qi stagnation is the cause if the constipation occurs when the person is upset; qi deficiency is implicated if a person feels fatigued after a bowel movement. In blood or yin deficiency, the stools are exceptionally dry, making them difficult to pass.

Frequent passing of clear urine indicates kidney deficiency; if the urine is concentrated (dark yellow), it is a sign of heat. Bed-wetting can also occur in kidney deficiency; in children, the cause of the bed-wetting is usually emotional. Lack of urination can arise from very deficient kidneys or occur due to severe heat, blood stagnation, or a stone.

Whatever its cause, lack of urination is a life-threatening condition, since the body can quickly become overwhelmed by its own toxins. In general, pale urine is a sign of cold, dark urine is a sign of heat, and cloudy urine is a sign of dampness. Sharp pain or blood in the urine can result from a stone or heat in the urinary bladder. Blood without pain could be a sign of cancer.

Use of Lifestyle Factors in Traditional Chinese Medicine Diagnosis

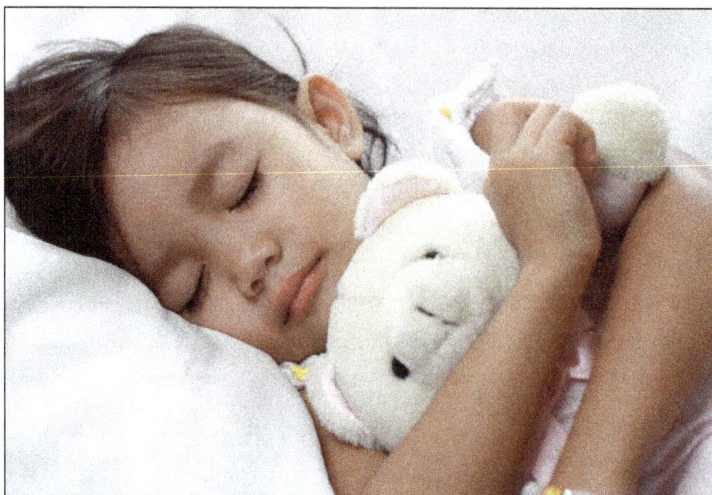

As Western and Eastern doctors will tell you, the amount of sleep you get affects your health.

Lifestyle factors can help a practitioner make a diagnosis in Chinese medicine. These factors, such as the amount of sleep you get each night, play a role in your overall health.

The practitioner should also evaluate your past medical history to get a clearer picture of your health.

Thirst, Appetite and Taste

No desire for fluids at all is a sign of excess cold, while a desire for small amounts of hot liquids can indicate deficiency cold from yang depletion. A craving for large amounts of water is a sign of excess heat. If a person has a dry mouth and wants small amounts of water, it is a sign of deficiency heat due to depleted yin.

If dampness is present, a person may want to drink but is unable to do so and may even vomit small amounts of water. A person with an excessively strong appetite may have stomach heat; he or she might even eat a lot but remain thin.

A person who has an appetite but no desire to eat could have stomach yin deficiency. In this case, the deficiency heat causes a false appetite, but the deficiency in stomach yin itself prevents true hunger. On the other hand, a complete lack of appetite indicates spleen qi deficiency; when the person does eat, he or she often feels bloated or tired afterward. When the appetite is low and the person has an aversion to oily foods, the cause could be damp heat in the liver and gallbladder.

Another set of diagnostic indicators unique to Chinese medicine is the presence of various tastes in the mouth. For example, a bitter taste in the mouth indicates heat, usually in the heart, liver, or gallbladder. A sweet taste can occur with damp heat in the spleen, and a salty taste can arise from a deficiency in the kidneys. A sour taste is associated with heat in the liver or food stagnation in the stomach, while a complete lack of taste can occur with spleen qi deficiency.

Sleep

A restful night's sleep depends on a healthy balance of yin and yang. The yin and blood are the aspects of the heart that provide a solid foundation for the mind and spirit. If yin and blood are deficient, yang will be out of control. Yang is fire and activity and is kept within normal ranges by cool and calm yin. When yin is deficient, it can't control yang, and too much heat and activity results, producing such symptoms as restlessness and insomnia.

On the other hand, if qi or yang is insufficient, the person experiences an overabundance of yin, leading to fatigue and excessive sleepiness. A person who has difficulty falling asleep but then sleeps soundly may have a deficiency of heart blood. Difficulty staying asleep can be a sign of deficient heart yin. The deficiency heat disturbs sleep. Insomnia that is accompanied by a bitter taste in the mouth and angry dreams is associated with liver fire, while sleeplessness due to irritability and sexual dreams can be a result of heat due to kidney yin deficiency.

A person who wakes up easily, is forgetful, and experiences heart palpitations can have a pattern of insufficient heart blood and spleen qi. In children, crying at night can often be due to heat in the heart or liver. A practitioner also attempts to determine whether a person gets too much sleep, since this could be due to qi or yang deficiency. If the person claims his whole body feels heavy, especially when the weather is rainy, the excessive sleep is caused by dampness.

Lifestyle and Medical History

Many imbalances are due to the patient's lifestyle. It is very difficult to treat a case of cold dampness in the spleen successfully in a person who eats a quart of ice cream every day - no matter how much ginseng and ginger the person consumes. Ice cream is classified as a cold, damp food. On the other hand, the same person can assist the healing process by consuming hot soups containing ginger root and pepper.

Foods are also strong medicines with their own hot or cold energies, and selecting the proper foods for a given body type or disease pattern is an important part of the healing process. Similarly, a person who walks around barefoot in the winter might complain about frequent colds. This person would be better off dressing in warm clothing, rather than trying to stimulate the immune system.

A complete medical history is just as important in traditional Chinese medicine as it is in Western medicine. Important clues might be uncovered that could shed light on the cause of current problems. It's important to note the use of any prescription medication, since a patient's symptoms could be due to side effects of these medications.

Gynecologic Signs and Symptoms

A female patient is always asked about her menstrual cycle, since it can provide abundant information about the condition of the internal organs and vital substances. A cycle that is longer than normal might be a sign of blood deficiency or cold stagnation, while a short cycle can occur with heat.

A scanty menstrual flow with light-colored blood is associated with deficiency of qi and blood, while a strong flow with dark color can be a sign of excess heat. Cramping before the menstrual flow is a symptom of excess, while cramping after the flow begins is a sign of deficiency. Blood clots with sharp pains occur with blood stagnation. If there is no cycle at all, the primary causes are qi and blood deficiency or stagnation.

Tongue Diagnosis

"Tongue diagnosis" is a practice long used in traditional Chinese medicine. According to the principles of TCM, analyzing the appearance of an individual's tongue can provide a greater understanding of his or her overall health.

Once a tongue diagnosis is completed and other aspects of the patient's health are evaluated, the practitioner may recommend treatment with such therapies as acupuncture, acupressure, herbal medicine, food therapy, and massage.

Tongue Exam to Assess Health

In TCM, it's thought that different areas of the tongue reflect the health of five corresponding organ systems: liver, lung, spleen, heart, and kidney. TCM is based on the theory that all of the body's organs mutually support each other and that – in order to achieve optimal health – an individual's organs must be in balance.

Although it's been used in TCM for many years, tongue diagnosis and its validity as a medical assessment tool haven't been thoroughly explored in scientific studies. Still, preliminary research suggests that tongue diagnosis shows promise as a means of evaluating certain measures of health in patients with conditions like rheumatoid arthritis and breast cancer.

Tongue diagnosis should not be used as a substitute for standard medical care or to diagnose potential health problems.

Factors considered in Tongue Assessment

During tongue diagnosis, TCM practitioners usually examine the tongue coating, shape, and color. Tongue diagnosis also involves examining specific areas on the tongue. Here's a look at how these issues are addressed in a typical tongue diagnosis:

Color: A light red color indicates that an individual's vital energy (also known as "qi") is strong. Changes in tongue color, meanwhile, are said to signal chronic illness.

For example, pale coloring in the tongue is thought to indicate an issue with the pancreas and/or digestive function, while purple coloring is said to arise from blockages in the flow of Qi.

Shape: Normal tongue shape is neither too thick nor too thin; the tongue body is smooth with no cracks. In general, changes in tongue shape are thought to reflect chronic illness affecting the blood, bodily fluids, or qi.

Changes in tongue shape may include a swollen or puffy tongue (said to be another indicator of problems with the pancreas and digestive function), cracks in the tongue (a possible sign of imbalance in the heart organ, an issue associated with insomnia and memory troubles), and curling at the sides of the tongue (thought to indicate liver qi stagnation).

Coating: Although the tongue coating is usually thin and white, a pale yellow and slightly thicker coating at the back of the tongue may also be normal.

In addition to reflecting the health of the spleen and stomach, tongue coating also provides an indication of acute illness (such as colds). For instance, a peeled or absent tongue coating may result from kidney yin deficiency, an issue associated with conditions like low back pain and tinnitus.

Here are some key points to keep in mind if you're thinking of undergoing a tongue diagnosis:

- Some disorders don't show up on the tongue. It should also be noted that TCM practitioners do not rely on tongue diagnosis alone in evaluating a patient's health.

- In most cases, the tongue is examined for no longer than 15 seconds at a time. Extending the tongue for longer may cause changes in tongue shape and color (two crucial elements of tongue diagnosis).

- Before receiving a tongue diagnosis, you should avoid food and beverages that might discolor your tongue (including coffee, beets, and foods made with artificial food coloring). Consumption of vitamin C may also affect your tongue coloring.

- If you use a tongue brush as part of your oral hygiene routine, discontinue use of the brush for at least a full day prior to your tongue diagnosis.

Pulse Diagnosis

The use of touch in making a diagnosis in Chinese medicine is integral. The art of touch in traditional Chinese medicine is highly sophisticated and includes the palpation of areas of pain and diagnostic points and the reading of the patient's pulse.

Regions and Methods for Taking Pulse

Regions for Taking Pulse

Cunkou, also known as "Qikou" (opening of Qi), is the usual pulse taking region, refers to pulsation of radial artery on the wrist. Cunkou is located on the pulsation of the lung meridian where Qi and blood in the lung meridian flows by. Besides, Qi and blood from all viscera circulates through the lung and converges over Cunkou. The lung meridian starts from the middle Jiao and converges with the spleen meridian. Since the spleen and the stomach are the sources of Qi and blood and function as postnatal base of life, Cunkou can reflect the conditions of the gastric Qi. On the other hand, the lung meridian is the meridian from where all the other meridians begin and end their circulation, because the circulation of Qi and blood in all the twelve meridians starts from and ends at the lung meridian, finally converging over Cunkou. That is why Cunkou can reflect the conditions of all viscera, Qi, blood and meridians in the body.

Pulse over Cunkou is divided into three parts: Cun, Guan and Chi, the part slightly below the styloid process of radius is Guan pulse, the part anterior the Guan pulse is the Cun pulse, and the part posterior the guan pulse is the Chi pulse. Both hands have three divisions of pulse, i. e. Cun pulse, Guan pulse and Chi pulse. So altogether there are six divisions of pulse.

Clinically the correspondence of Cunkou pulse and the viscera is decided according to the description in Neijing, that is the upper pulse (Cun pulse) corresponds to the upper part of the body and the lower pulse (Chi pulse) corresponds to the lower part of the body:

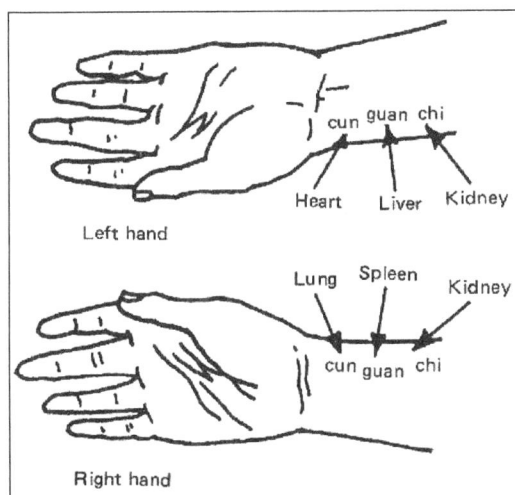

- The left Cun pulse is corresponding heart and Tanzhong (the part between the breasts).

- The left Guan pulse is corresponding liver and gallbladder.

- The left Chi pulse is corresponding kidney and the lower abdomen. The right Cun pulse is corresponding lung and thorax.

- The right Guan pulse is corresponding spleen and stomach.

- The right Chi pulse is corresponding the kidney and the lower abdomen.

Such a theory about the relationship between the Cunkou pulse and the corresponding viscera is significant in clinical diagnosis. However, the application should be flexible and based on the synthetic analysis of the data obtained from the four diagnostic methods.

Methods for Taking Pulse

The following points should be borne in mind in taking pulse:

Time: Early morning is the ideal time for taking pulse because the conditions of the pulse are not affected by food and other activities. However, this requirement is difficult to fill in clinical practice. To ensure accurate pulse taking, the patient should rest for a while to tran- quilize the heart and breath before pulse taken. The pulse should be taken at least for one minute each time in order to correctly examine the conditions of the pulse.

Normal and calm breath: Normal and calm breath means that the doctor keeps his or her own breath quiet to examine the pulse of the patient and calculate the beat of the pulse according to his or her own cycle of exhalation and inhalation. Healthy people breathe 16 - 18 times one minute under normal conditions. And the pulse beats 4 - 5 times in a cycle of exhalation and inhalation, about 60 - 90 beats per minute.

Posture: The patient sits erect or lies in their back and the forearms stretches out naturally to the level of the heart. The wrist is put straight, the palm turns over and the fingers are relaxed to extend the Cunkou region and enable Qi and blood to flow freely.

Arrangement of fingers: The three fingers of doctor are put at the same level and slightly arched to press the pulse with the belly of the fingers. The middle finger presses on the guan pulse, the index finger presses on the region anterior the guan pulse (distal to the heart region), and the ring finger on the chi pulse posterior to the guan pulse (proximal to the heart region). The arrangement of the fingers is made according to the conditions of the patient's arm. In diagnosing diseases in children, "one finger is used to press just the guan pulse". It is unnecessary to divide the pulse into three parts in this case.

General pressure and single pressure: General pressure means to press the pulse with three fingers to distinguish the conditions of Cun, Guan and Chi pulses on both hands. Single pressure means to examine the pulse on one hand with just one finger to differentiate the states of Cun, Guan and Chi pulses. Clinically these two methods are used according to the pathological conditions in question.

Lifting, pressing and searching: Lifting, pressing and searching refer to flexible pressure of pulse in order to distinguish the conditions of pulse.

Lifting (Ju) means light pressure; pressing (An) means heavy pressure; and searching (Xun) means mobile moderate pressure which is used to look for the most obvious region of the pulse. In the procedure of diagnosis, doctors should pay attention to the use of these three methods to distinguish the variations of pulse.

Exam the pulse conditions: The pulse conditions are felt by doctor's fingers. The examination of pulse conditions means to distinguish the features of pulse according to the position of pulse, the rhythm of pulse, the shape of pulse and the strength of pulse.

Normal Pulses

Normal pulse refers to the pulse conditions of the healthy people.

1. The shape of the normal pulse: The normal pulse is neither floating nor sunken, neither fast nor slow, sensible with moderate pressure, usually beating 4 - 5 times in a cycle of breath (about 60-90 beats per minute), gentle in sensation, powerful in rebounding, moderate in size, regular in beating and varying with physical activities and environmental changes.

2. The characteristics of the normal pulse: The normal pulse is marked by gastric qi, spirit and root. Gastric qi means that the pulse is located at the middle, neither floating nor sunken, and regular in beating, moderate in size, gentle in sensation and floating. Spirit means that the pulse is soft, powerful and rhythmic. Root means that the chi pulse is powerful and constantly beating under heavy pressure.

    Gastric qi, spirit and root are three basic features of the normal pulse which complement each other and cannot be separated. Simultaneous appearance of the three reflects strong functions of the viscera and sufficiency of qi and blood.

3. Main factors to affect the normal pulse: The normal pulse may vary with physiological and psychological factors in the human body and the environmental factors outside.

Age, sex and body shape: The pulse is usually small and fast in children, smooth and slippery in young people, taut and hard in old people, moderate and powerful in men, soft and thin in women, slippery and fast in pregnant women, sunken and thin or soft and thin in obese people, floating and large in lean people, long in tall people and short in small people.

Daily life and psychological factors: The pulse appears slippery, fast and powerful after movement, eating and drinking of wine, weak with hunger, taut in anger and irregular in fright.

Seasonal, alternation of day and night and geographical factors: The pulse appears slightly taut in spring, slightly full in summer, slightly floating in autumn and slightly sunken in winter; slightly floating and powerful in the daytime and slightly sunken, thin and slow in night; sunken and energetic among the people in the north and soft among the people in the south.

Besides, the changes of the anatomic position of the radial artery may shift the pulse normally at the Cunkou region to the dorsum of the hand from the chi region, known as oblique flying pulse. The pulse, shifted to the back of the Cunkou region, is called ectopic radial pulse.

All the factors above mentioned may affect the conditions of the pulse. However, if the pulse still keeps gastric Qi, spirit and root, it is still the normal pulse.

Abnormal Pulses

There are five elements of abnormal pulse diagnosis:

- Position: Deep or superficial,
- Frequency: Rapid or slow,
- Morphology: Wide or thin, long or short, hard or soft, fluent or not,
- Strength: Strong or weak,
- Rhythm: Regular or irregular.

According to Depth

Superficial Pulse (Fu Mai)

- Features: Sensible under light pressure, weak and constant beating under heavy pressure. It is marked by superficial beating.
- Clinical significance: Floating pulse indicates external syndrome, floating and powerful pulse signifying external excess syndrome while floating and weak pulse manifesting external asthenia syndrome. Floating pulse can also be seen in internal asthenia syndrome due to consumption of essence and blood in chronic disease and external floating of deficient Yang.

Deep Pulse (Chen Mai)

- Features: Sensible only under heavy pressure.
- Clinical significance: Indicating internal syndrome. Sunken and powerful pulse signifies excess internal syndrome, while sunken and weak pulse shows deficient internal syndrome.

According to Frequency

Slow pulse (Chi Mai)

- Features: Less than 60/min (<4 beats in a breath cycle).
- Clinical significance: Indicating cold syndrome. Slow and powerful pulse signifies excess cold syndrome, while slow and weak pulse shows deficient cold syndrome. Such a pulse condition is also seen in internal excess heat syndrome due to internal accumulation of pathogenic heat. Athletes with slow pulse are in a normal condition.

Moderate Pulse (Huan Mai)

- Features: The pulse is moderate and powerful, beating 4 times in a cycle of breath; or moderate and sluggish, beating 4 times in a cycle of breath (60-70/min).

- Clinical significance: Normal or indicating dampness and weakness of the stomach and spleen.

Rapid Pulse (Shuo Mai)

- Features: More than 90/min (>5 - 6 times in a breath cycle).

- Clinical significance: Indicating heat syndrome. Rapid and powerful pulse signifies excess heat syndrome, while rapid and weak pulse shows deficient heat syndrome. Such a pulse condition is also seen in the syndrome due to external floating of deficient Yang.

Swift Pulse (Ji Mai)

- Features: The pulse beats over 7 times in a breath cycle (>140/min).

- Clinical significance: Indicating loss of control of hyperactive yang, declination of kidney Yin and near depletion of primordial Qi.

This pulse is so rapid (twice the normal speed) that it is easily detected; the acute febrile disease involves an easily measured high temperature and is usually subject of pathogen testing. Consumptive conditions with such high pulse rates are generally under emergency medical care.

According to Morphology

Surging Pulse (Hong Mai)

- Features: Surging pulse is marked by wide size and full content, beating like roaring waves and sensibility under light pressure and surges as well as sudden flowing and ebbing.

- Clinical significance: Indicating exuberant internal heat.

Thin Pulse (Xi Mai)

- Features: The pulse is as thin as a thread, weak and quite sensible under pressure.

- Clinical significance: Indicating deficiency of both Qi, Yin and blood, various overstrain and diseases due to pathogenic dampness.

According to Length

Long Pulse (Chang Mai)

- Features: The pulse surpasses the range of cun, guan and chi regions.

- Clinical significance: Indicating yang syndrome, heat syndrome and excess syndrome.

Short Pulse (Duan Mai)

- Features: The pulse appears shorter than the normal content of cun, guan and chi regions.

According to Hard or Soft

Slippery Pulse (Hua Mai)

- Features: The pulse is beating freely and smoothly like the movement of beads of an abacus.

- Clinical significance: Indicating retention of phlegm and fluid, dyspepsia and excess heat. Such a pulse condition is also seen among young and strong and pregnant people.

Wiry Pulse (Xuan Mai)

- Features: Wiry pulse appears straight, energetic and hard like the feeling of pressing the string of a violin.

- Clinical significance: Indicating disorders of the liver and gallbladder, pain syndrome and retention of phlegm and fluid.

Tense Pulse (Jin Mai)

- Features: Tense pulse appears like the pulling of a rope and flicks the finger when pressed.

- Clinical significance: Indicating cold syndrome, pain syndrome and retention of food.

Soft/Soggy Pulse (Ru Mai)

- Features: Superficial, soft, weak and thin, become weak under heavy pressure. Clinical significance: Indicating Qi and blood deficirncy, and dampness syndrome.

This pulse is similar to the fine and weak pulses. The thready pulse sensation felt on light touch gives the impression of being easily moved, as if floating on water; hence, it tends to indicate spleen Qi deficiency with accumulation of dampness.

According to Fluency

Astringent/Choppy Pulse (She Mai)

- Features: The pulse is beating in an inhibited way like scraping a piece of bamboo.
- Clinical significance: Astringent and powerful pulse indicates qi stagnation and blood stasis; astringent and weak pulse signifies lack of essence and insufficiency of blood.

According to Strength

Weak Pulse (Xu Mai)

- Features: Weak pulse is marked by weak beating of the pulse at all the cun, guan and chi regions.
- Clinical significance: Indicating deficirncy syndrome, usually seen in asthenia of both qi and blood, especially in Qi asthenia.

Feeble Pulse (Ruo Mai)

- Features: Feeble pulse is deep and thin as well as sensible and weak under heavy pressure.
- Clinical significance: Indicating declination of both Qi and blood.

Indistinct Pulse (Wei Mai)

- Features: Indistinct pulse is very thin and soft, almost insensible under pressure.
- Clinical significance: Indicating extreme deficiency of qi and blood as well as declination of yang qi.

Scattered Pulse (San Mai)

- Features: Rootless, arrhythmic and disappearing under pressure.
- Clinical significance: Indicating depletion of primordial qi, visceral essence at the verge to exhaust and external floating of deficient yang.

These are cases where the patient is critically ill, perhaps near death; such patients are normally hospitalized (or sent home to die) and their diagnosis is usually well-established. The pulse only tells that the patient is severely debilitated; it diffuses on light touch and is faint with heavy pressure.

Hollow Pulse (Kou Mai)

- Features: Floating, large and hollow like the leaf of scallion.

- Clinical significance: Indicating loss of blood and impairment of yin.

Powerful Pulse (Shi Mai)

- Features: Powerful pulse is marked by powerful sensation of pulse beating at cun, guan and chi regions under superficial, moderate and heavy pressure.

According to Rhythm

Rapid and Irregular Pulse, (Cu Mai)

- Features: Rapid and intermittent pulse beats fast with irregular intermittence.

- Clinical significance: Fast and powerful pulse indicates hyperactivity of Yang, heat, Qi stagnation, blood stasis and retention of phlegm and food; fast and weak pulse signifies weakness of visceral Qi and insufficiency of blood.

This pulse is so rapid (twice the normal speed) that it is easily detected; the acute febrile disease involves an easily measured high temperature and is usually subject of pathogen testing. Consumptive conditions with such high pulse rates are generally under emergency medical care.

Slow and Irregular Pulse, (Jie Mai)

- Features: The pulse beats slowly with irregular intermittence.

- Clinical significance: Slow, intermittent and powerful pulse indicates predominance of Yin, Qi stagnation, retention of phlegm, and blood stasis; while slow, intermittent and weak pulse signifies declination of qi and blood.

Regularly Irregular Pulse (Dai Mai)

- Features: The pulse beats slowly with regular and longer intermittence.

- Clinical significance: Indicating declination of visceral Qi and asthenia of primordial Qi.

Eight Principles of Diagnosis

According to TCM, illness arises as a result of specific yin-yang imbalances of the Functional Entities. The functional entities are:

- The Five Fundamental Substances: Qi, Xue (Blood), Jinye (Body Fluids), Jing (Essence), and Shen (Spirit).

- Zang-fu: A Wu Xing cycle of 5 zang organs, 6 fu organs, and their functions.

- Jing-luo: The channels or meridians through which qi flows.

The functional entities are responsible for performing the five cardinal functions that maintain health within the body. They are: Actuation, Warming, Defense, Containment, and Transportation.

If there is an imbalance within the any of the functional entities, they will not be able to perform their cardinal functions, and as result, illness may arise.

Oriental Medicine does not evaluate an illness purely based on the symptoms a person is showing, but rather, on complex patterns of disharmony in the body.

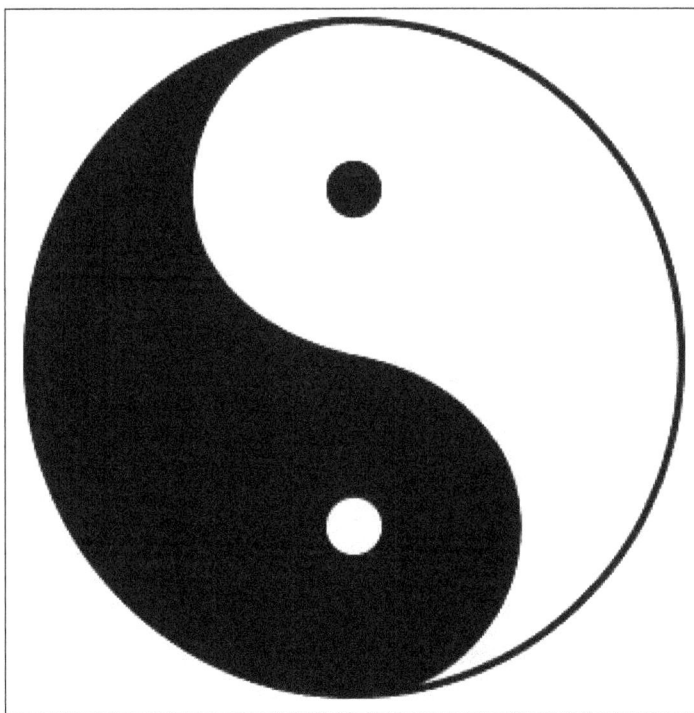

At the most basic level, these patterns are determined by eight principles, which measure either an excess (vacuity) or deficiency (stagnation) of qi in one the entities.

The process of determining the actual pattern of diagnosis begins with an evaluation of bing according to the notion of the eight principles. The eight principles describe the basic qualities of a disease. This notion refers to four pairs of mutual opposites. The eight principles are:

1. Yin: Yin, along with yang is the most general classification for pattern diagnosis and it describes the relationship between the other three pairs of the Principles. Generally speaking, yin is Cold.

2. Yang: Yang, along with yin is used to describe the relationship between the other three pairs of the Principles. For example, Heat is Yang.

3. Interior: Interior describes diseases that manifest themselves in the Zang-fu organs or deep inside the body, such as qi, blood, and bone marrow. More broadly, it used to describe diseases that cannot be classified as Exterior.

4. Exterior: Exterior describes diseases that manifest themselves on surface of the body, such hair, skin, nails, and meridians. Its clinical features include body chills, fever, aversion to cold temperatures and winds, a weak pulse, and headaches.

5. Heat: Heat describes the absence of an aversion to Cold. If paired with an Exterior pattern, its symptoms can include a rapid pulse, fever, body chills, dehydration, and a sore throat. If paired with an Interior patter, its symptoms can include a preference for cold drinks, clear urine, and a slow pulse.

6. Cold: Cold describes an aversion to cold. If paired with an Exterior pattern, its symptoms can include body aches, a tense pulse, fever, body chills, and headaches. If paired with an Interior patter, its symptoms can include nausea, stomach pain, vomiting, and diarrhea.

7. Deficiency: Deficiency is used to describe a vacuity in qi, blood (Xue), or body fluids (Jinye). Depending on how it relates to Interior/Exterior and Cold/Heat, it can manifest as constipation, having a small appetite, dizziness, and slow pulse.

8. Excess: Excess is generally classified as any disease that can't be identified as a Deficiency pattern. Usually, it means that one of the Six Excesses is present. Depending on how it relates to Interior/Exterior and Cold/Heat, it can manifest as quick pulse, sweaty palms, and sharp stomach pains.

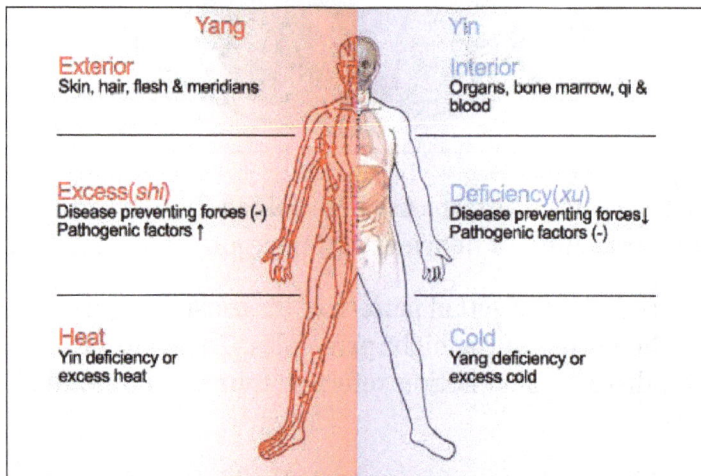

After a basic diagnosis of the diseases is given via the eight principles, the diagnostic continues and focuses on more specific conditions. After evaluating the present symptoms, a person's condition is further evaluated as to how the specific entities (qi, meridians, Zang-fu, etc.) are affected.

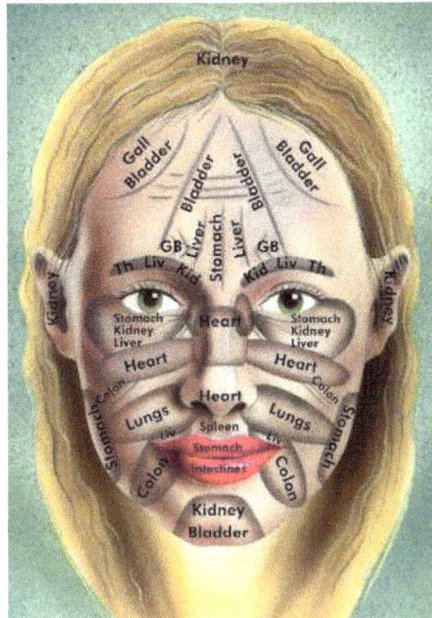

Four Pillars of Diagnosis

There are four methods of diagnostics in Traditional Chinese Medicine, which are often referred to as the Four Pillars of Diagnosis. They are:

- Inspection: Inspection or "looking" focuses on visual analysis of the face, skin features, and particularly, the tongue. In TCM, the surface of the tongue corresponds to particular zang-fu organs and can reveal a lot about a particular disease. Therefore, the tongue diagnosis is considered a cornerstone practice in the diagnostic process.

- Auscultation: Auscultation refers to the analysis of particular sounds. In TCM, there are five major types of sounds: shouting, laughing, singing, weeping, and groaning. Auscultation analysis extends to olfaction, which analyzes the smell of body odor, even though sound and smell are consider to be separate senses in the West.

- Palpation: Palpation refers to analysis by feeling, particularly the wrist pulse, abdomen, and meridians points. The techniques for doing are complex and can years to learn.

- Inquiry: Inquiry refers to analysis by asking questions about the person's past health and habits. Traditionally, this included 10 questions, which ranged from diet to sleep pattern.

After recognizing a particular pattern of disharmony, a doctor will prescribe treatment based on the diagnosis that was given. The treatment can include the more common practices of Traditional Chinese Medicine, such as herbal medicine, acupuncture, and tui na massage, but also less common practices, such as cupping.

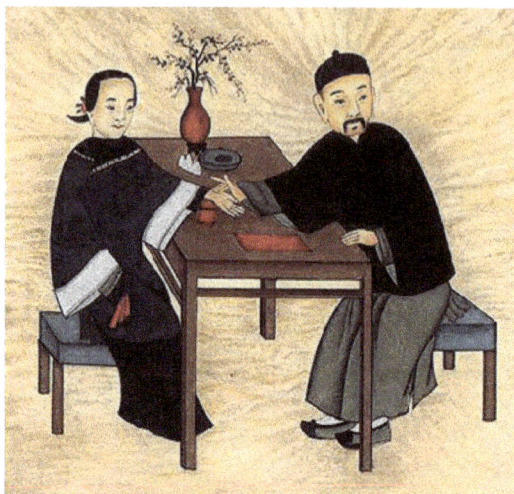

Yin and Yang

Yin and Yang is one of the most fundamental concepts in Traditional Chinese Medicine (TCM), as it is the foundation of diagnosis and treatment. The earliest reference to Yin and Yang is in the I Ching (Book of Changes) in approximately in 700 BC. In this work, all phenomena are said to be reduced to Yin-Yang.

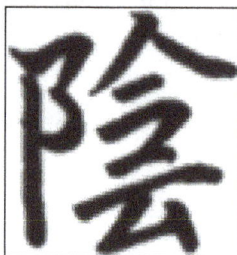

Yin

Translations

- Female, Passive,

- Negative Principle in Nature,

- The Moon,

- Shaded Orientation,

- North or Shady Side of a Hill,

- South of a River.

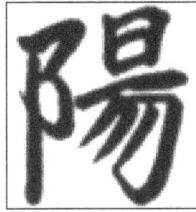

Yang

Translations

- Positive, Active,

- Male Principle in Nature,

- South or Sunny Side of a Hill,

- North of a River.

Four Main Aspects of Yin and Yang Relationship

- Yin-Yang are opposites: They are either on the opposite ends of a cycle, like the seasons of the year, or, opposites on a continuum of energy or matter. This opposition is relative, and can only be spoken of in relationships. For example: Water is Yin relative to steam but Yang relative to ice. Yin and Yang are never static but in a constantly changing balance.

- Interdependent: Can not exist without each other: The Tai Ji (Supreme Ultimate) diagram shows the relationship of Yin & Yang and illustrates interdependence on Yin & Yang. Nothing is totally Yin or totally Yang. Just as a state of total Yin is reached, Yang begins to grow. Yin contains seed of Yang and vise versa. They constantly transform into each other. For Example: no energy without matter, no day without night. The classics state: "Yin creates Yang and Yang activates Yin".

- Mutual consumption of Yin and Yang: Relative levels of Yin Yang are continuously changing. Normally this is a harmonious change, but when Yin or Yang are out of balance they affect each other, and too much of one can eventually weaken (consume) the other. Four possible states of imbalance:

  ○ Preponderance (Excess) of Yin.

  ○ Preponderance (Excess) of Yang.

- ◦ Weakness (Deficiency) of Yin.

- ◦ Weakness (Deficiency) of Yang.

- • Inter-transformation of Yin and Yang: One can change into the other, but it is not a random event, happening only when the time is right. For example: Spring only comes when winter is finished.

Twenty-four Hour Yin Yang Cycle

12 PM corresponds to Utmost Yang, while 12AM corresponds to Utmost Yin.

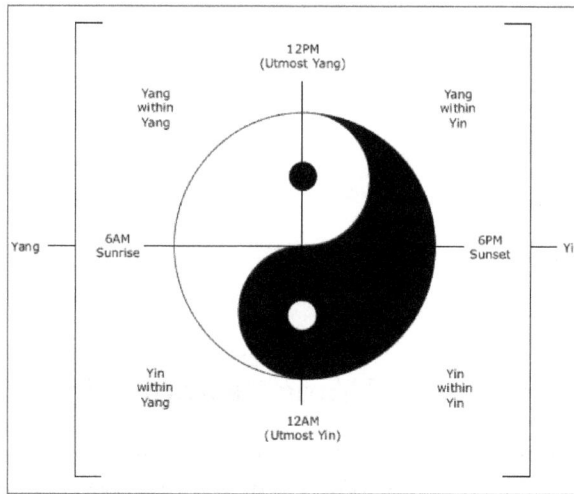

General Qualities of Yin and Yang

Yin	Yang
Darkness	Light
Moon	Sun
Feminine	Masculine
Shade	Brightness
Rest	Activity
West (Sunset = Yin)	East (Sunrise = beginning of Yang)
North	South
Earth	Heaven
Right	Left
Flat (like Earth)	Round (like Heaven)
Matter	Energy
More material/dense	Non-material, rarefied

These transform into one another. They are 2 states of a continuum.i.e. - Liquid water (Yin) heat - vapor (Yang) - cools - liquid (Yin).

Yin	Yang
Produces form	Produces energy
Grows	Generates
Substantial	Non-substantial
Matter	Energy
Contraction	Expansion
Descending	Rising
Below	Above
Water	Fire

Yin and Yang in Medicine

All physiological processes, signs and symptoms can be reduced to Yin-Yang.

In general, every treatment modality aims to:

- Tonify Yang;

- Tonify Yin;

- Disperse excess Yang;

- Disperse excess Yin.

(In practice, depending on the condition, strategies may be combined, for example: disperse excess Yin & tonify Yang).

Yin and Yang and the Six Pathogenic Factors

Yin	Yang
-	Wind
Cold	Heat
Dampness	Dryness
-	Summerheat

Yin and Yang and the Human Body

Yin	Yang
Front (chest-abdomen)	Back
Body	Head
Interior (organs)	Exterior (skin, muscles)
Below waist	Above waist
Anterior-medial	Posterior-lateral

ventral surface of the trunk and limbs	back and dorsal surface of the limbs
Structure	Function
Blood/Body Fluids	Qi
Conservation/storage	Transformation/change
Yin Organs: Heart, Lung,	Small Intestine, Lg. Intestine
Liver, Spleen, Kidney,	Gall Bladder, Stomach, Bladder
Pericardium	San Jiao
"Solid Organs"	"Hollow Organs"

Front and Back

Front is more soft and vulnerable (Yin). Back contains spine that holds ribs: protection. When human depicted as crouching, back receives sun (Yang) and front faces the earth (Yin), is in shade and is protected.

All Yang channels (except the Stomach channel) flow on the dorsal or dorsolateral surface of the trunk and limbs. They carry Yang energy and protect the body from pathogenic factors. Yin channels flow on the anterior or anteromedial surface of the trunk and limbs.

Body and Head

Yang channels either end or begin on the head. Acupuncture points on the head can be used to raise Yang energy. When Yang energy is not cooled by Yin, it may rise to the head, causing signs such as red face and eyes. The head is easily affected by Yang pathogens such as heat and wind. The chest and abdomen (Yin) areas are more easily affected by Yin pathogens such as Cold and Dampness.

Interior and Exterior

The exterior of the body such as the skin and muscles is more Yang. The exterior protects body from attack by external pathogenic influences such as Cold, Wind, etc. The classics state: "Yang is on the outside and protects Yin".

Below the Waist and Above the Waist

Below waist - closer to earth (Yin). Above, closer to Heaven (Yang).

Upper part more affected by Yang pathogens, i.e. wind.

Lower part more affected by Yin pathogens, i.e. cold damp.

Anterior/Medial and Posterior/Lateral Surface of the Limbs

Yin channels flow on anterior-medial aspect of trunk/limbs. Yang channels flow on posterior-lateral aspect of trunk/limbs.

Structure and Function

Structure = Something substantial, i.e. Matter (Yin).

Function = Something insubstantial, action, energy (Yang).

All parts of the body have a structure (a physical form), and a function (their activity).

However, all is relative. Even within the Yang category of function, there are Yin functions (i.e. storage, conservation) and Yang functions, i.e. transformation, transportation, digestion, excretion.

Within the Yin category of form there are Yin forms ("solid") and Yang forms ("hollow").

Blood, Body Fluids and Qi

Qi is Energy, more Yang.

Blood = Denser and more material (therefore Yin).

But note that "Xue" (blood) not exactly like our concept of Blood. More like "thicker" form of Qi.

There are several types of Qi. Each is relatively more Yin or Yang.

Ancestral QI (more Yin, more slow moving. Moves in long slow cycles).

Ying Qi (more Yang than Ancestral Qi, moves with Blood with which it is closely related). Ying is more Yin than Wei Qi.

Wei Qi the most Yang form of Qi. Circulates in the exterior in the daytime to protect us from pathogenic influences, and regulates opening/closing of pores.

Conservation/Store (Yin) and Transformation/Change (Yang)

Yin Organs store Blood, Body Fluids, Essence, etc.

Yang Organs constantly transform, transport and excrete the products of digestion.

Solid and Hollow Organs (Zang Fu)

Yin Organs are "Solid": Constantly active, involved in production and storage of the body's vital Substances (Qi Blood, Body Fluids, Essence).

Yang Organs are "Hollow": Receive and circulate but do not store, involved in digestion, transformation, excretion.

Yin and Yang in Pathology

Clinical signs and symptoms can be interpreted via Yin-Yang theory. When Yin Yang are in dynamic balance and relating harmoniously, there are no symptoms to observe. When Yin and Yang are out of balance, they become separated.

For example (Actual symptoms depend on specific pathologies, which Organ involved, etc.):

- When Yin does not cool and nourish Yang, then Yang rises (headaches, red face, sore eyes, sore throats, nosebleeds, irritability, manic behavior).

- When Yang does not warm and activate Yin (cold limbs, hypo-activity, poor circulation of blood, pale face, low energy).

Yin	Yang
Deficiency	Excess
Hypo-activity	Hyperactivity
Chronic disease/gradual onset	Acute disease/rapid onset
Slowly changing symptoms	Rapid pathological changes
Quiet, lethargy, sleepiness	Restlessness, insomnia
Wants to be covered	Throws off bedclothes
Lies curled up	Lies stretched out
Cold limbs and body	Hot limbs and body
Pale face	Red face
Weak voice, no desire to talk	Loud voice, talkative
Shallow, weak breathing	Coarse breathing
No thirst/wants warm drinks	Thirst esp. for cold drinks
Copious, clear urine	Scanty, dark urine
Loose stools (fluids not transformed)	Constipation (damage to fluids by heat)
Clear, copious secretions	Thick, sticky white/yellow secretions
Excessive moisture	Excessive dryness (throat, skin, eyes etc.)
Degenerative disease	Inflammatory disease
Pale tongue, white coat	Red tongue, yellow coat
Empty pulse	Full pulse

In Practice

Although Yin-Yang is essential for understanding symptoms and signs, the above list of signs is too general. We need to distinguish further to get exact diagnosis. i.e. which TCM Organs involved, which pathogens involved, which channels involved.

Structure and Function - Without structure, function could not occur. Without function, structure would be meaningless.

Mutual Consumption of Yin and Yang - Balance of Yin & Yang is constantly changing. Yin & Yang mutually consume each other.

Four Different Situations

For additional signs and symptoms for general deficiency and excess of Yin and Yang,

Yin	Yang
Excess of Yin	Excess of Yang
Deficiency of Yin	Deficiency of Yang

- Excess of Yin i.e., when excess Cold in the body consumes the Yang (heat). This is an Excess Cold (Full Cold) condition.

- Excess of Yang i.e., when excess Heat (from Exterior or Interior of body) consumes Body Fluids, leading to Dryness or even Heat. This is an Excess Heat (Full Heat) condition.

- Deficiency of Yin (Consumption of Yin) i.e., when the body's Yin energy is depleted, an apparent excess of Yang results, leading to feelings of "empty heat" (mild but very specific heat symptoms, i.e., flushed cheeks, afternoon fever, sweating at night, heat in extremities. This is Deficiency Heat (Empty Heat) condition (i.e., a condition of deficiency and heat), also called "False Fire".

- Deficiency of Yang (Consumption of Yang) - When body's Yang energy is spontaneously deficient - an apparent excess of Yin results, leading to various symptoms involving cold and hypo-activity Deficiency of Yang can also occur after an Excess Cold condition has damaged Yang. This is an Deficiency Cold (Empty Cold) condition (i.e., a condition of deficiency and cold).

Yin	Yang
Excess of Yin (Full Cold)	Excess of Yang (Full Heat)
Excess of Yin is primary aspect	Excess of Yang is primary aspect
Yin is in true excess	Can eventually cause deficiency of Yin
Can eventually cause deficiency of Yang	
Yin	Yang
Deficiency of Yang (Consumption of Yang)	Deficiency of Yin (Consumption of Yin)
(Empty Cold)	(Empty Heat of "False Fire")
Decrease of Yang energy is primary aspect	Deficiency of Yin is primary aspect
Yin only apparently in excess	Yang only apparently in excess

Inter-transformation of Yin and Yang in Medicine

In medicine also, Yin and Yang transform into one another, but only when conditions are right. The right moment determined by internal qualities of the given situation or phenomenon. In clinical practice, the above principle is very important.

Disease is prevented by living a balanced lifestyle, like the examples below:

- Excessive work (Yang) without rest leads to deficiency of Yin energy.

- Excessive consumption of cold food (Yin) leads to deficiency of body's Yang energy.

- Smoking (adding heat 'Yang' into Lungs) leads to deficiency of Yin of Lungs (and eventually Kidneys).

The principle is observable in pathological changes seen in disease, like the examples below:

- Exterior cold (cold weather) can invade body and can change to heat (sore throat).

- Deficiency of Spleen Yang can lead to Excess Interior Dampness (Yin), because the Spleen Yang is unable to properly transform fluids.

References

- Causes-of-disease-in-chinese-medicine: agelessherbs.com, Retrieved 17 March, 2019

- Traditional-chinese-medicine-causes-of-illness3, chinese, natural-medicine, wellness: howstuffworks.com, Retrieved 13 February, 2019

- Traditional-chinese-medicine-diagnosis, chinese, natural-medicine, wellness: howstuffworks.com, Retrieved 3 May, 2019

- Tongue-diagnosis-in-traditional-chinese-medicine: verywellhealth.com, Retrieved 15 January, 2019

- Eight-principles-of-diagnosis-in-tcm: amcollege.edu, Retrieved 28 April, 2019

- Yin-yang, get, foundations-chinese-medicine: sacredlotus.com, Retrieved 23 June, 2019

Chapter 6

Therapies in Traditional Chinese Medicine

There are various therapies which are used within traditional Chinese medicine. A few of them are Chinese cupping, Chinese tuina massage, gua sha, acupressure, qi gong, tai chi and Chinese dietary therapy. This chapter has been carefully written to provide an easy understanding of the varied facets of these therapies in traditional Chinese medicine.

Chinese Cupping

Cupping is the term applied to a technique that uses small glass cups or bamboo jars as suction devices that are placed on the ski to disperse and break up stagnation and congestion by drawing congested blood, energy or other humors to the surface. In dry cupping, the therapist will simply place the suction cups on the skin. In wet cupping, the practitioner will make a small incision on the skin and then apply the suction cup to draw out small amounts of blood.

There are several ways that a practitioner can create the suction in the cups. One method involves swabbing rubbing alcohol onto the bottom of the cup, then lighting it and putting the cup immediately against the skin. Suction can also be created by placing an inverted cup over a small flame, or by using an alcohol-soaked cotton pad over an insulating material (like leather) to protect the skin, then lighting the pad and placing an empty cup over the flame to extinguish it. Flames are never used near the skin and are not lit throughout the process of cupping, but rather are a means to create the heat that causes the suction within the small cups.

Once the suction has occurred, the cups can be gently moved across the skin (often referred to as "gliding cupping). Medical massage oils are sometimes applied to improve movement of the glass cups along the skin. The suction in the cups causes the skin and superficial muscle layer to be lightly drawn into the cup. Cupping is much like the inverse of massage – rather than applying pressure to muscles, it uses gentle pressure to pull them upward. For most patients, this is a particularly relaxing and relieving sensation. Once suctioned, the cups are generally left in place for about ten minutes while the patient relaxes. This is similar to the practice of Tui Na, a traditional Chinese medicine massage technique that targets acupuncture points as well as painful body parts, and is well known to provide relief through pressure.

The side effects of cupping are fairly mild. Bruising should be expected, but skin should return to looking normal within 10 days. Other potential side effects include mild discomfort, skin infection, or burns. However, a trained health professional will apply an antibiotic ointment and bandage to prevent an infection.

Philosophy behind Pain and Cupping

"Where there's stagnation, there will be pain. Remove the stagnation, and you remove the pain." The old Chinese medical maxim holds that pain results from the congestion, stagnation, and blockage of Qi, or vital energy, vital fluids, lymph, phlegm, and blood. If pain is the essence of disease, then suffering is a result of obstructed or irregular flow in the body. Chinese cupping is therefore a method of breaking up the blockage to restore the body's natural flow of energy.

Cupping Combined with Acupuncture

Generally, cupping is combined with acupuncture in one treatment, but it can also be used alone. The suction and negative pressure provided by cupping can loosen muscles, encourage blood flow, and sedate the nervous system (which makes it an excellent treatment for high blood pressure). Cupping is used to relieve back and neck pains, stiff muscles, anxiety, fatigue, migraines, rheumatism, and even cellulite. For weight loss and cellulite treatments, oil is first applied to the skin, and then the cups are moved up and down the surrounding area.

Like acupuncture, cupping follows the lines of the meridians. There are five meridian lines on the back, and these are where the cups are usually placed. Using these points, cupping can help to align and relax qi, as well as target more specific maladies. By targeting the meridian channels, cupping strives to 'open' these channels – the paths through which life energy flows freely throughout the body, through all tissues and organs, thus providing a smoother and more free-flowing qi (life force). Cupping is one of the best deep-tissue therapies available. It is thought to affect tissues up to four inches deep from the external skin. Toxins can be released, blockages can be cleared, and veins and arteries can be refreshed within these four inches of affected materials. Even hands, wrists, legs, and ankles can be 'cupped,' thus applying the healing to specific organs that correlate with these points.

Other Benefits of Chinese Cupping

This treatment is also valuable for the lungs, and can clear congestion from a common cold or help to control a person's asthma. In fact, respiratory conditions are one of the most common maladies that cupping is used to relieve.

Cupping's detoxifying effect on skin and circulatory system is also significant, with a visible improvement in skin color after three to five treatments. Cupping removes toxins and improves blood flow through the veins and arteries. Especially useful for athletes is cupping's potential to relieve muscle spasms.

Cupping also affects the digestive system. A few benefits include an improved metabolism, relief from constipation, a healthy appetite, and stronger digestion. A report noted cupping as an effective alternative method of treating acne, pain, facial paralysis, cervical spondylosis, and herpes zoster.

As health practitioners and researchers continue to study the benefits of cupping, this traditional alternative care technique will gain further acceptance and wider practice across holistic healthcare centers in the U.S. as an effective treatment for a wide variety of ailments.

Chinese Tuina Massage

Tuina or tui-na massage originated in ancient China and is believed to be the oldest system of bodywork. It's one of the four main branches of traditional Chinese medicine, along with acupuncture, qi gong, and Chinese herbal medicine.

It's based on the theory that imbalances of qi, which is the body's vital life force or energy, can cause blockages or imbalances that lead to symptoms such as pain and illness.

Tuina massage stimulates the flow of qi to promote balance and harmony within the body using many of the same principles of acupuncture. It's similar to acupuncture in the way it targets specific acupoints, but practitioners use fingers instead of needles to apply pressure to stimulate these points. Tuina massage is often used in combination with acupuncture.

The philosophy and principles of tuina massage are based on traditional Chinese medicine, which focuses on emotional and physical components of a person's well-being, as well as aspects such as climate, relationships, and diet. The underlying philosophy of tuina massage is that true health is achieved when one has found harmony and balance inside the self and their environment. The goal of tuina massage is to create harmony in the yin and yang of the body by getting rid of blockages and disturbances that manifest as illness, disease, and emotional issues.

Similar to acupuncture, tuina massage uses the same energetic meridians and acupoints to balance the qi and blood in your body, leading to better health. Qi that's flowing incorrectly can cause blockages, such as poor blood circulation in the affected area. The main therapeutic goal of tuina massage is to remove the energetic blocks that are causing qi stagnation.

Technique

During a session, practitioners use oscillating and pressure techniques that differ in force and speed. Tuina massage can be done as a stronger deep-tissue massage or a more gentle, energetic treatment.

Some techniques are more yin, which is more gentle, passive, and meditative. The yang approach is more active, dynamic, and physical, creating more intense sensations by stimulating deep blockages and knots.

The practitioner massages the muscles and tendons and uses manipulation techniques to realign the body. Passive joint movements are used to restore function to muscles and joints. Depending on your practitioner as well as your specific needs, various techniques will be used in a session. To enhance the effects of the treatment, herbal poultices or compresses, lotions, and salves are used.

Tuina massage uses massage techniques such as acupressure, myofascial release, and reflexology. Sometimes, techniques that are common to osteopathy and chiropractic, such as stretching and joint mobilizations, are also used.

There are eight basic techniques used in tuina massage:

- Palpating (mo)
- Rejoining (jie)
- Opposing (duan)
- Lifting (ti)
- Pressing (an)
- Kneading (mo)
- Pushing (tui)
- Holding (na)

Other techniques include:

- Rolling: This is used for injuries such as sprains and strains.
- One-finger technique: This is one-finger stimulation of acupressure points.
- Nei gung: This is a full-body manipulation technique.

What does it Treat?

Tuina massage can be used to treat specific health concerns or areas in the body. Since tuina massage is considered to be an alternative treatment, it's essential that you talk to your doctor before using it to treat any medical condition.

Tuina massage can be used to treat pain and illness, or to maintain good health. The technique is effective in reducing stress, encouraging relaxation, and deepening sleep. It's often used for conditions and injuries related to the musculoskeletal and nervous systems.

Here are some conditions tuina massage can treat:

- Neck and back pain;

- Musculoskeletal disorders;

- Premenstrual syndrome;

- Fatigue and insomnia;

- Carpal tunnel;

- Headaches;

- Arthritis;

- Osteoporosis;

- Stress;

- Digestive conditions;

- Respiratory conditions.

Benefits

While some of the research is preliminary and ongoing, there's plenty of evidence to back the effectiveness of tuina massage in treating health conditions.

1. Boosts blood circulation: One of the main intentions of tuina massage is to boost blood circulation by stimulating the body's energy flow.

A small 2015 study indicates that yi zhi chan tuina manipulation on BL 56 acupoint is effective in improving circulation. In this study, manipulation using medium force for 10 minutes was found to be more effective than treatments using light or heavy force for shorter amounts of time.

2. Reduces neck pain: Tuina massage relieves neck pain and the accompanying tension, tightness, and irritation.

A 2018 study concluded that tuina massage is a cost-effective option for reducing pain in people with chronic neck pain. People who received six tuina treatments within three weeks reduced the intensity of their neck pain more than people who had no treatment.

3. Relieves low back pain: Tuina massage can relieve lower back pain, especially when treatment is paired with core exercises. Researchers in a 2016 study found that tuina massage was more effective when combined with core stability exercises in people with low back pain.

People who did tuina massage alone had higher rates of back pain at follow-up compared to people who incorporated core exercises to their treatment.

4. Treats depression: Focusing on whole-body healing is essential for people with depression, since the causes can be both physical and emotional. Studies concluded that tuina massage has a therapeutic effect on depression. It was shown to be significantly more effective in reducing depression than conventional treatments.

5. Promotes healthy lactation: Tuina massage is used to encourage postpartum lactation. The results of a 2012 study showed that tuina massage on breasts increased the quantity of lactation compared to women who received only conventional treatment.

Though no significant difference was found between the groups in terms of delaying the decrease of prolactin levels, researchers believe tuina massage could have a positive effect in this area. It could help new mothers produce greater quantities of milk more quickly.

6. Treats osteoarthritis: The therapeutic benefits of tuina massage extend to alleviating symptoms of osteoarthritis. According to a small 2011 study shows, it improves muscular tension of the flexor and extensor muscles in people with knee osteoarthritis. The treatment used gun, an, na, and ca maneuvers. The patients received treatments three times per week over the course of nine months. Patients saw improvement in pain, stiffness, and function.

7. Eases carpal tunnel syndrome: According to this 2010 study, tuina massage can relieve symptoms from carpal tunnel syndrome. People with carpal tunnel syndrome who received warm-needling acupuncture in addition to tuina massage showed significantly more improvements than people who were treated using hormone block therapy and medication.

8. Treats musculoskeletal disorders: Tuina massage is often used to improve function and reduce pain affecting the joints, bones, and muscles. Meta-analysis points to the effectiveness of tuina massage in treating musculoskeletal disorders. The technique was shown to be effective in relieving pain, especially compared to traction, medication, and physical therapies. Evidence to support better function wasn't as strong as pain reduction.

9. Benefits foot issues from diabetes: Tuina massage can be beneficial for people with diabetes who have foot issues. A 2018 study found that tuina massage combined with

a Chinese medicine foot bath was therapeutically beneficial for people with early-stage diabetic foot.

People who received tuina massage and a foot bath in addition to conventional medicine showed significant improvements compared to people who received only conventional medicine.

10. Improves quality of life in cancer patients: Tuina massage is a viable option for people with cancer who want to manage symptoms related to the disease and its conventional treatment.

A 2016 meta-analysis assessed the effect of tuina massage on improving symptoms and quality of life for people with cancer. The meta-analysis also looked at the effects of:

1. Acupuncture,

2. Tai chi,

3. Qi gong,

4. Traditional Chinese medicine five-element music therapy.

When combined with acupuncture, tuina massage was effective in improving quality of life in people with terminal cancer. Tuina massage was also shown to be effective in relieving stomach discomfort.

Though tuina massage shows promise as a therapy to treat people with cancer, more in-depth research is needed, as many of the studies had limitations.

Side Effects

Tuina massage is a safe treatment and is generally well-tolerated. However, remember that it's not a gentle or relaxing massage, and you may feel some discomfort during or after a session. Slight bruising is possible.

It's not recommended for people who have fractures or are prone to fractures, vein inflammation, or any type of open wound. It's also not recommended for people with previous chronic back issues, such as ankylosing spondylitis.

Gua Sha

Skin Scraping (Gua Sha) is one of the traditional Chinese natural therapies. It is based on the skin theory of traditional Chinese medicine: by using tools such as jade, ox horn or cupping jars with liniment on, scraping and rubbing repeatedly the relevant parts of the skin, to dredge the channel, and activate blood circulation to dissipate blood stasis.

Regular Skin Scraping is helpful to adjust the qi, relieve fatigue, and improve one's immune system.

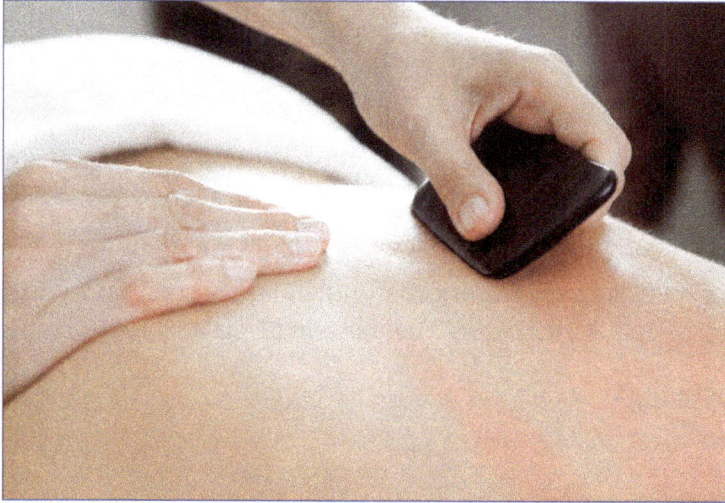

Skin Scraping therapy has a long history. It originated in the Paleolithic Age. When people were sick, out of instinct, they rubbed or hit some parts of the body with hands or stones, and sometimes it really alleviated the disease's symptoms. Through long-term practice and accumulation, the method of curing the diseases with stones was formed. It gradually developed into a therapy through the support of the scientific system of Chinese medicine. The Chinese character (sha) comes from (meaning sand), and the latter first refers to a symptom. As after scraping the patients' skin, there might be lots of red, dark purple or dark blue spots like sand, so the therapy gradually earned the name "Gua Sha."

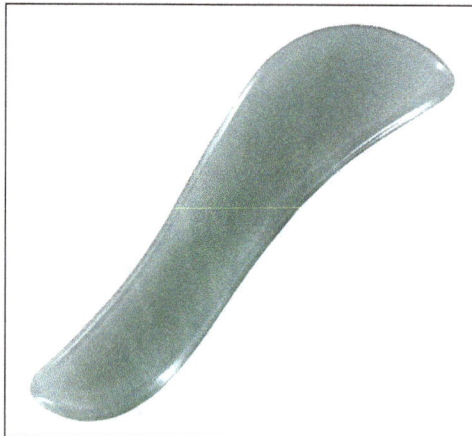

The principle of Skin Scraping is very easy to understand: through scraping the meridian points, good stimulation is created. This can help the yingqi and weiqi play their roles, engorge the meridian points and improve local circulation, so that the potential for disease resistance and immune function are enhanced. In fact, early in the Ming Dynasty, the physician Zhang Fengkui described the reason, pathogenesis and the symptom of Sha in his Book about Diseases in the Summertime. In his view, the toxic factor enters the body through mouth, nose and pores, and damages the health. It turns fierce as it goes deep in the body and accumulates more and more. Skin Scraping therapy uses tools to scrap the surface of the meridian points till the emergence of red spots on the skin. Through sweating, the toxins of Sha will be excreted, and the purpose of healing is achieved.

In addition to traditional scraping therapy, skin scraping health therapy, scraping therapy to lose weight, scraping therapy to dispel freckle and other new therapies has appeared to meet the need of the modern time. Especially the skin scraping health therapy is developed from the traditional therapy. Due to the development of the modern technology, the tools of scraping are becoming more suitable for the scraping of every parts of the body. The techniques also become more reasonable. Combined with the techniques of massage, hitting at meridian points and acupuncture, Skin Scraping has become the massage without direct hand touching, acupuncture without needle in the body, and cupping without cupping jars.

Under the pressure of fast-paced life, modern people face with the problems of poor health, so the natural therapy of Skin Scraping is beginning to attract many people's attention again. It has become the choice of more and more people to keep their health.

Gua sha may reduce inflammation, so it's often used to treat ailments that cause chronic pain, such as arthritis and fibromyalgia, as well as those that trigger muscle and joint pain. Gua sha may also relieve symptoms of other conditions:

1. Hepatitis B: Hepatitis B is a viral infection that causes liver inflammation, liver damage, and liver scarring. Research suggests that gua sha may reduce chronic liver inflammation.

One case study followed a man with high liver enzymes, an indicator of liver inflammation. He was given gua sha, and after 48 hours of treatment he experienced a decline in liver enzymes. This leads researchers to believe that gua sha has the ability to improve liver inflammation, thus decreasing the likelihood of liver damage.

2. Migraine headaches: If your migraine headaches don't respond to over-the-counter medications, gua sha may help. In one study, a 72-year-old woman living with chronic headaches received gua sha over a 14-day period. Her migraines improved during this time, suggesting that this ancient healing technique may be an effective remedy for headaches.

3. Breast engorgement: Breast engorgement is a condition experienced by many breast-feeding women. This is when the breasts overfill with milk. It usually occurs in the first weeks of breastfeeding or if the mother is away from the infant for any reason. Breasts become swollen and painful, making it difficult for babies to latch. This is usually a temporary condition.

In one study, women were given gua sha from the second day after giving birth up until leaving the hospital. The hospital followed up with these women in the weeks after giving birth and found that many had fewer reports of engorgement, breast fullness, and discomfort. This made it easier for them to breastfeed.

4. Neck pain: Gua sha technique may also prove effective for remedying chronic neck pain. To determine the effectiveness of this therapy, 48 study participants were split into two groups. One group was given gua sha and the other used a thermal heating pad to treat neck pain. After one week, participants who received gua sha reported less pain compared to the group that didn't receive gua sha.

5. Tourette syndrome: Tourette syndrome involves involuntary movements such as facial tics, throat clearing, and vocal outbursts. According to a single case study, gua sha combined with other therapies may have helped to reduce symptoms of Tourette syndrome in the study participant.

The study involved a 33-year-old male who had Tourette syndrome since the age of 9. He received acupuncture, herbs, gua sha, and modified his lifestyle. After 35 once-a-week treatments, his symptoms improved by 70 percent. Even though this man had positive results, further research is needed.

6. Perimenopausal syndrome: Perimenopause occurs as women move closer to menopause. Symptoms include:

- Insomnia

- Irregular periods

- Anxiety

- Fatigue

- Hot flashes

One study, however, found that gua sha may reduce symptoms of perimenopause in some women. The study examined 80 women with perimenopausal symptoms. The intervention group received 15 minute gua sha treatments once a week in conjunction with conventional therapy for eight weeks. The control group only received conventional therapy.

Upon completion of the study, the intervention group reported greater reduction of symptoms such as insomnia, anxiety, fatigue, headaches, and hot flashes compared to the control group. Researchers believe gua sha therapy might be a safe, effective remedy for this syndrome.

Side Effects of Gua Sha

As a natural healing remedy, gua sha is safe. It's not supposed to be painful, but the procedure may change the appearance of your skin. Because it involves rubbing or scraping skin with a massage tool, tiny blood vessels known as capillaries near the surface of your skin can burst. This can result in skin bruising and minor bleeding. Bruising usually disappears within a couple of days.

Some people also experience temporary indentation of their skin after a gua sha treatment. If any bleeding occurs, there's also the risk of transferring bloodborne illnesses with gua sha therapy, so it's important for technicians to disinfect their tools after each person.

Avoid this technique if you've had any surgery in the last six weeks. People who are taking blood thinners or have clotting disorders aren't good candidates for gua sha.

Acupressure

Acupressure is often called acupuncture without the needles. Instead of needles, acupressure involves the application of manual pressure (usually with the fingertips) to specific points on the body.

According to the principles of traditional Chinese medicine, the body has invisible lines of energy flow called meridians. There are thought to be at least 14 meridians connecting our organs with other parts of the body. Acupuncture and acupressure points lie on those meridians.

If the flow of energy (also called "chi" or "qi") is blocked at any point on a meridian, it's thought to cause various symptoms and health conditions anywhere along the meridian. That's why a practitioner may apply pressure to an acupressure point on the foot to relieve a headache.

There is no consensus on how acupressure might work. Some theorize that the pressure may promote the release of natural pain-relieving chemicals in the body, called endorphins. Another theory is that the pressure may somehow influence the autonomic nervous system.

Uses

Most people try acupressure for the first time to manage symptoms of a condition, such as:

- Cancer-related fatigue,
- Headache,
- Menstrual cramps,
- Motion sickness,
- Muscle tension and pain,

- Nausea or vomiting after surgery or chemotherapy,

- Nausea and vomiting during pregnancy and morning sickness,

- Stress management.

Benefits

There's currently a lack of studies exploring the effectiveness of acupressure. Still, there's some evidence suggesting that wrist acupressure may help to relieve pain after a sports injury. Researchers examined the effects of three minutes of acupressure, three minutes of sham acupressure, or no acupressure in athletes who had sustained a sports injury on the same day.

At the study's end, acupressure was found to be effective in reducing pain intensity compared to sham acupressure or no acupressure. There was no change in anxiety.

Acupressure may help to ease nausea and vomiting in those with chemotherapy-induced nausea and vomiting. Researchers analyzed the results of three previously published trials and found that acupressure (using finger pressure or an acupressure wristband) decreased nausea, vomiting, and retching.

In a report scientists analyzed 22 previously published clinical trials on acupuncture or acupressure for the induction of labor and found no clear benefit in reducing the cesarean section rate.

Typical Acupressure Session

Acupressure is often administered by an acupuncturist, with the person receiving the acupressure sitting or lying down on a massage table. Acupressure can also be self-administered. While it's best to consult an acupuncturist for proper instruction, acupressure is generally done by using the thumb, finger, or knuckle to apply gentle but firm pressure to a point. The pressure is often increased for about 30 seconds, held steadily for 30 seconds to two minutes and then gradually decreased for 30 seconds. It's typically repeated three to five times.

The point "P6" can be found by turning the arm so that the palm is facing up. Place the thumb at the center of the crease of the wrist (where the hand meets the wrist) and then position it two finger widths away from the crease towards the elbow. The point is between the two large tendons.

Side Effects and Safety

Acupressure should never be painful. If you experience any pain, tell your therapist immediately. After an acupressure session, some people may feel soreness or bruising at acupressure points. You may also feel temporarily lightheaded. Pressure should be gentle over fragile or sensitive areas, such as the face.

If you have a condition such as osteoporosis, recent fracture or injury, cancer, easy bruising, a bleeding disorder, heart disease, uncontrolled blood pressure, diabetes, or are using anticoagulant or antiplatelet medications such as warfarin, you should speak to your doctor before trying acupressure.

If you are pregnant, you should speak to your care provider before trying acupressure. Acupressure typically isn't done on the abdomen or certain points on the leg or low back during pregnancy.

Acupressure shouldn't be done over open wounds, bruises, varicose veins, or any area that is bruised or swollen.

Qi Gong

Qigong is an ancient Chinese health care system that integrates physical postures, breathing techniques and focused intention.

Being an art of self-training both body and mind as well as sending forth external qi, Qigong, created by the Chinese people in the long process of life, labor and fight against diseases, protecting and strengthening health and prolonging life. It is one of the gems in the treasure-house of China's cultural heritage as well as component part of traditional Chinese medicine.

Qigong has a long history and diverse schools. As the "internal qi" of qigong and the "external qi" emitted by Qigong masters are invisible and inaudible to ordinary people, Qigong is commonly considered to be mysterious and profound.

Qigong is an art and skill to train qi. To be exact, it is a method by which the practitioner gets physical and mental self-exercise through bringing into play his subjective initiative. To achieve this aim, the practitioner must associate his mind, postures and breathing and act on the whole. On one hand, it actively self-regulates the functional activities of the organism and maintains a dynamic equilibrium. On the other hand, it enables the body to produce an "energy-storing" reaction, reduce energy consumption and increase energy accumulation, producing the effects of regulating yin and yang, dredging the channels and collaterals and emitting external qi.

Taiji Quan of Qigong

Taijiquan is a style of qigong. It is graceful, relaxed, slow, and fluid, like a slow-motion dance. Unlike some qigong methods that exercise specific systems or parts of the body - nervous system, endocrine system, heart, kidneys - Taijiquan is a whole body, whole mind exercise. It treats health systemically, restoring the body to its original "program", uncorrupted by stress, pollution, and disease.

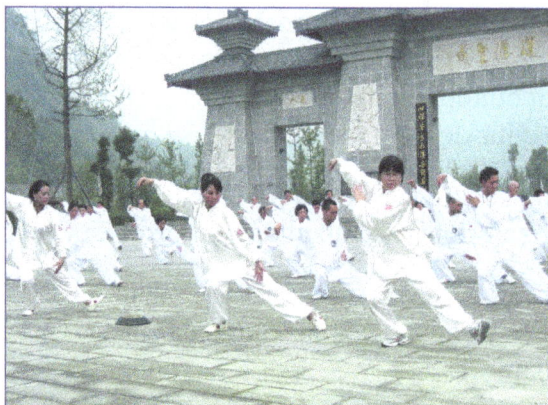

Modern Researches on Qigong

Influence of Qigong on the Neuromuscular System

When the training practice reaches the Qigong state, the electroencephalograph dynamic process research finds: the peak frequency under Qigong state diminishes in accordance with the variations of time, the dynamic variance falls and the fluctuation of the peak amplitude diminishes. It can be seen that the EEG stability is enhanced and the ordering degree is improved. Meanwhile, the rhythm of the frontal region is strengthened, indicating that the control of the brain over the activities of the internal organs and the incretory glands is somewhat strengthened.

Under Qigong tranquilization, various components of the body-sensory evoked potential in the experiment display various degrees of restraint, the late components being the most obvious in particular, manifested by descent of wave amplitude or distortion of undulate form. Some components have disappeared. The researchers hold that this is because in the process of Qigong, through auto-regulation the reticular structure is made to produce an ascending restraint over the sensory transmission. In addition, in the process of Qigong tranquilization the sense perception of electrical stimulation reduces or disappears, denoting that the response to sensual stimulation is reduced.

The determination of the skin electrical potential of the acupoints Feishu and Mingmen finds that the skin electrical potential is reduced in the process of the training practice. During the training practice, the Dantian and other regions' body surface temperature rises. Meanwhile, it can also be observed that when the training practice reaches the tranquilization state the heart rate slows down, while the volume of the ear lobe blood vessels increases, the two presenting a negative correlation. These discoveries show that Qigong dirigation can reduce the excitability of the sympathetic nervous system in the vegetative nerves and raise the excitability of the parasympathetic system.

When the training practice has reached the tranquilization state, the relaxation degree of the skeletal muscles is increased and the electromyogram presents single electrical potential pattern or electrical quiescence.

Influence of Qigong on the Respiratory System

During the training practice, the frequency of respiration obviously decreases, the depth of respiration deepens, the pulmonary ventilation volume reduces, tidal volume increases, the carbon dioxide component in the expiratory air and alveolar air increases while the oxygen component reduces. These show that in the process of the training practice respiration is in a spontaneous weakening state.

Influence of Qigong on the Digestive System

Qigong dirigation can increase the peristaltic frequency of the stomach and intestines, strengthen their contraction and cause the hyperfunction of the intestinal gurgling sound, promoting the secretion of gastric juice. These effects also indicate that the training practice lays the cerebral cortex in a specific qigong state and regulates the functional condition of the vegetative nerves, manifested as the rise of the excitability of the vagus nerve and the fall of the excitability of the sympathetic nerve, thus regulating the movement and secretory function of the stomach and intestines.

Meanwhile, the respiration exercise of qigong is dominated by diaphragmatic movement. The deep and profound abdominal respiration can increase the amplitude of the diaphragmatic movement by 3-4 times, changing the intra-abdominal pressure and promoting the peristalsis of the stomach and intestines.

Three Key Elements of Qigong

Regulation of Body in Qigong (Postures)

It is essential to assume suitable postures in qigong dirigation. Correct postures are the preconditions to guarantee smooth respiration and induce mental relaxation and tranquilization. The theory that "if the postures are not correct, the flow of qi can not be smooth; if the mind is not concentrated, qi will be in disorder" shows the importance of the regulation of body.

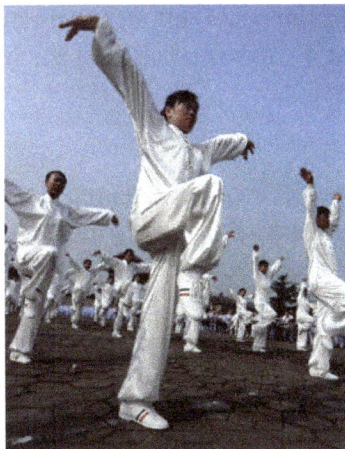

Plain Sitting Posture

Sit up straight on a square stool, with the trunk and thighs, thighs and shanks in an angle of 90° respectively at the suitable height, the knees separated shoulder-width apart, the feet firmly placed on the floor, the hands naturally placed on the knees or thighs, the lower jaw slightly drawn in, the shoulders relaxed and the chest slightly drawn in, the mouth and eyes slightly closed, the tip of the tongue raised against the hard palate and a smile on the face.

Free Knee-crossing Posture

Sit up straight on a wood bed with the legs crossed in the shape of the Chinese word (eight), sitting naturally with the legs crossed, the hands placed on the knees or with the fingers interlocked before the lower abdomen, palms facing upward. The postures of the upper part of the body, head and upper limbs are the same as in Plain Sitting Posture.

Supine Lying Posture

Lie on the back on a wood bed with the upper part of the body cushioned slightly higher presenting a sloping position, with the legs straightly stretched, the hands placed against the sides of both legs or on the lower abdomen with one palm over the other (palms facing downward). The requirements of the head are the same as in Plain Sitting Posture.

Standing Posture

Take the Tri-round-style Standing Stump for an example. Stand with the feet parallel to each other 3-4 foot-widths apart (the space can be regulated in accordance with the height of the stance), head and neck right straight, the lower jaw slightly drawn in, the chest slightly drawn in and back erect, the hip relaxed and knees bent, the eyes looking straight ahead or slightly closed; the arms presenting an embracing gesture with the five fingers of each hand naturally separated and lightly bent as if holding a ball, the fingertips of one hand pointing at those of the other, about 30 cm apart, palms facing inward; the mouth naturally closed, the tongue tip raised against the hard and a smile on the face.

Walking Posture

Stand still for 2-3 minutes, then left foot takes a step forward first, with the heel touching the ground first, the upper part of the body and the hands swinging to the right, inhale through the nose and exhale through the mouth; when the left foot fully touches the ground, take the right foot one step forward with the heel touching the ground first, the upper of he body and the arms swinging to the left, inhale through the nose and exhale through the mouth. Walk forward step by step as described above and end the exercise after walking for about half an hour.

Regulation of Breathing in Qigong (Respiration)

The regulation of breathing is the regulation and exercise of respiration. It is a very important link in training qi, an essential method to cause genuine qi in the human body to accumulate, initiate and circulate. The regulation of breathing not only can achieve the effects of regulating the qi and blood and massaging the internal organs of the organism but is also helpful to mental tranquilization and physical relaxation. The breathing regulation methods commonly adopted are as follows:

Natural Respiration Method

Without exertion of mindwill, breathe naturally.

1. Orthodromic Abdominal Respiration Method: This refers to the method of respiration in which the diaphragm descends with the abdomen bulging out in inhalation and the diaphragm rises with the abdomen drawn in exhalation.

2. Counter-abdominal Respiration Method: Contrary to the above method, this refers to the method of respiration in which the abdomen is drawn in inhalation and bulges out in exhalation.

3. Pausing-closing Respiration Method: This refers to the respiration method which requires pausing and closing qi for a little while after each inhalation (exhalation) and then exhale (inhale).

4. Nose-inhaling and Mouth-exhaling Method: This refers to the respiration method to inhale through the nose and exhale through the mouth.

Regulation of Mind in Qigong (Mind-will)

The key link in the regulation of mind is to, through exertion of mindwill, concentrate the mind, get rid of all stray thoughts, replace myriads of thought, thus gradually induce into tranquilization and enter a state of void. This is, namely, the so-called "training the mind to return to void". This is the most essential exercise in qigong dirigation. The effect of the training practice is mainly determined by the degree of tranquilization. It is comparatively difficult for beginners to tranquilize. The tranquilizing methods commonly adopted are as follows:

Mind Concentration Method

The mind is highly concentrated on certain part of the body, certain acupoint or certain object outside the body, usually concentrated on Dantian. The concentration should be obscure, without any forceful exertion, relaxed and natural, being just right.

Breathing Method

The mind is highly concentrated on respiration, concentrated only on the rise and fall of the abdominal respiration without the conduct of mindwill so as to form a unification of mindwill and qi and reach a tranquil state of mind.

Breach-counting Method

During the training practice, count silently the time of breath till the ear fails to hear, the eyes fail to see and the mind fails to think thus naturally reaching a tranquil state of mind.

Silent Reading Method

Read silently certain single word or phrase, for instance, the two words "relax" and "tranquilize", one word for exhalation and inhalation respectively. Its purpose is to replace the myriads of thoughts with one thought, replace all stray thoughts with the orthodox thought, gradually achieving a state free from stray thoughts and full of relaxation and joyousness, and comfortably reaching a tranquil state of mind.

Relaxation Qigong

Relaxation Qigong aims at regulating the whole body into a relaxed, comfortable and natural state through a step-by-step and rhythmical relaxation of all parts of the body coordinated by silently reading the relax - character formula. This maneuver has the functions of activating qi and blood, coordinating the internal organs, dredging the channels and collaterals, strengthening health, preventing and curing diseases.

- Preparations: Assume the standing, sitting or lying posture, with the tongue-tip raised against the hard palate, the eyes slightly drooping, the chest slightly drawn in and the back erect. Regulate breathing and concentrate the mind on Dantian.

- Tri-route relaxation Method: Tri-route Relaxation Method can be conducted on the foundation of reedy preparations.

- The Routes of Relaxation:

  ○ The first route: From the bilateral sides of the head, the bilateral sides of the neck, shoulders, upper arms, elbows, fore-arms, wrists and two hands to the ten fingers.

  ○ The second route: From the face, neck, chest, abdomen, two thighs, knees, shanks and two feet to the ten toes. The third route: From the back of the head, posterior nape, back, waist, posterior parts of both thighs, two popliteal fossae, two shanks and two feet to the soles of both feet.

- Method of Relaxation: First relax from the first route, going on from above to below. Having finished the first route, go on to the second and third routes. Generally, first focus on one location of one route and silently read the word "relax" (without any sound), then focus on the next location. Relax in this way link by link, route by routes, for 3-5 cycles altogether.

- Method of Local Relaxation: On the foundation of the relaxation of the three routes, the relaxation of certain part of the body can be carried out individually, such as the relaxation of the tension points and the locations of diseases and pains. Concentrate the mind on these locations and silently read the word "relax" for 20-30 times.

- Method of Whole-body Relaxation: Regard the whole body as a point to relax. One can read silently to effect a general one-shot relaxation from the head to the feet; or silently meditate to fly and fall from a high palace to relax or silently meditate to relax downwards continuously like water flowing along the routes of the Tri-route Relaxation Method.

Inner-nourishing Qigong

Inner-nourishing Qigong is a maneuver featured by the coordination of silent reading of words or phrases with respiration exercise. It has fairly food regulating effects on the functional activities of the nervous, circulatory and digestive systems.

- Preparations: The lying and plain sitting postures are the most suitable. Just before the training practice, drink a small amount of boiled water, loosen the clothes and belt, get rid of all stray thoughts and relax the mind.

- Coordinate silent reading of words, phrases or sentences with respiration exercise: The phrases or sentences for silent reading generally begin from three Chinese characters, to be increased gradually as time goes on, but ought not exceed ten characters at most. The content of the phrases or sentences are usually related to qigong dirigation, such as "tranquilize by myself", "I can relax and tranquilize", "sitting still leads to good health" and the like. The method of respiration is: inhale when silently reading the first word; hold one's breath when silently reading the middle word or words, the more the middle words are, the longer the time of holding breath is; exhale when silently reading the final word.

- Adopt abdominal respiration method: When inhaling, raise the tongue against the hard palate, naturally conduct qi to the lower abdomen and imagine in the mind "Qi sinks to Dantian". When exhaling, detach the tongue from the hard palate so as to allow air to go out naturally. During the practice of the above method, attention should be paid to inhalation rather than exhalation.

Tai Chi

Tai chi is an ancient Chinese tradition that, today, is practiced as a graceful form of exercise. It involves a series of movements performed in a slow, focused manner and accompanied by deep breathing. Tai chi, also called tai chi chuan, is a noncompetitive, self-paced system of gentle physical exercise and stretching. Each posture flows into the next without pause, ensuring that your body is in constant motion.

Tai chi has many different styles. Each style may subtly emphasize various tai chi principles and methods. There are variations within each style. Some styles may focus on health maintenance, while others focus on the martial arts aspect of tai chi. Tai chi is different from yoga, another type of meditative movement. Yoga includes various physical postures and breathing techniques, along with meditation.

Who can do Tai Chi?

Tai chi is low impact and puts minimal stress on muscles and joints, making it generally safe for all ages and fitness levels. In fact, because tai chi is a low-impact exercise, it may be especially suitable if you're an older adult who otherwise may not exercise.

You may also find tai chi appealing because it's inexpensive and requires no special equipment. You can do tai chi anywhere, including indoors or outside. And you can do tai chi alone or in a group class.

Although tai chi is generally safe, women who are pregnant or people with joint problems, back pain, fractures, severe osteoporosis or a hernia should consult their health care provider before trying tai chi. Modification or avoidance of certain postures may be recommended.

Why Try Tai Chi?

When learned correctly and performed regularly, tai chi can be a positive part of an overall approach to improving your health. The benefits of tai chi may include:

- Decreased stress, anxiety and depression,

- Improved mood,

- Improved aerobic capacity,

- Increased energy and stamina,

- Improved flexibility, balance and agility,

- Improved muscle strength and definition.

Some evidence indicates that tai chi may also help:

- Enhance quality of sleep;

- Enhance the immune system;

- Help lower blood pressure;

- Improve joint pain;

- Improve symptoms of congestive heart failure;

- Improve overall well-being;

- Reduce risk of falls in older adults.

Maintaining the Benefits of Tai Chi

While you may gain some benefit from a tai chi class that lasts 12 weeks or less, you may enjoy greater benefits if you continue tai chi for the long term and become more skilled.

You may find it helpful to practice tai chi in the same place and at the same time every day to develop a routine. But if your schedule is erratic, do tai chi whenever you have a few minutes. You can even practice the soothing mind-body concepts of tai chi without performing the actual movements when you are in a stressful situation, such as a traffic jam or a tense work meeting, for instance.

Chinese Dietary Therapy

In TCM there is no distinct difference between food and medicine, meaning that food itself can sometimes be all the medicine you need. Food is viewed as a powerful tool to help create and maintain wellness.

The basis of healthy eating in regards to TCM is filling most of the diet with fresh foods that are free from chemicals, preservatives, and over-processing. These foods are seen as the most vital, that is full of Qi.

Vegetables should be cooked only lightly to preserve beneficial enzymes and vitamins. People should eat according to their particular constitution with the largest meal of the day in the morning. Beans and grains should be soaked and properly cooked to allow for easy digestion. Not only is a healthy diet integral to optimal health, it is crucial to get physical and mental exercise as well as rest.

According to Chinese medicine, every food and herb has a nature, flavor, and organ system/meridian associated with it. The nature describes the effect of the food (or herbs) on the temperature of the body, while the flavor describes the taste.

Instead of viewing meals as a breakdown of proteins, carbohydrates (sugars), and fats, Chinese dietary therapy utilizes the flavors and natures of foods as a guide to a well-balanced meal. Learning how to utilize the nature and flavors of foods and herbs is really where the true healing capacity of this diet lays.

There is also the belief that the seasons have a profound impact upon our well-being, and eating according to the seasons can have great impacts on our health. We are immensely influenced by changes in the climate and we should learn to live and eat in balance with those changes.

Chinese diet therapy also focuses on a mentality that "like treats like." For example if woman had a particularly heavy menstrual cycle and was feeling fatigued, then eating some extra red meat or foods high in iron can help. If someone was struggling with pain in their joints, some bone broth can do the trick. Also foods that resemble parts of the body are often used to help support that specific part: walnuts for the brain, pomegranates for women's health.

Food as Everyday Medicine

There is a lot to learn when it comes to Chinese medicine and the Five elements, but even learning and incorporating the basics into your everyday life can have profound impacts. The main reason here is to observe your body and its patterns to learn what it needs to find balance. Some simple ideas are if you are feeling over heated- eat come cooling cucumbers, feeling bloated or have edema - cut down on your salt intake.

If you want to go deeper into Chinese dietary therapy it is advised that you see a Chinese medicine practitioner or acupuncturist. They will be able to figure out a pattern differentiation of your current constitution. This will usually be an explanation of where the body is out of balance in regards to the five elements (fire, earth, metal, water, wood) or organ systems (heart/small intestine, spleen/stomach, lung/large intestine, kidney/bladder, liver/gallbladder).

Once you have this information you will be able to make more informed decisions of what flavors, and natures of foods can nurture your body best.

5 Natures and 5 Flavors

Nature (Temperature)

The nature of foods and herbs describes the temperature changes that they cause within the body. (Warming foods help to move the blood and qi of the body to the surface and may cause sweating.) This not only has to do with the energetic properties and inherent temperature based-natures of the foods themselves but with how the foods are prepared or cooked (roasting, broiling, and heating equating to warm while iced and raw correspond to cold). Also plants that take longer to grow such as carrots, ginseng, cabbage or rutabaga are considered to be warmer foods then those that grow quickly such as cucumbers, radish, and lettuce.

Warming foods can help to stimulate body functions and raw food can help cool us down. Too much hot or warming foods can over stimulate our system while ingesting too many raw or cold foods can slow down our digestive processes. Like all things in Chinese medicine, it is about creating balance and finding harmony within your system, so eating a variety of warm and cool foods can help to create a well-balanced diet.

1. Hot

2. Warm

3. Neutral

4. Cool

5. Cold

Flavor

Understanding the five flavors of Chinese medicine is a very important part of its dietary therapy. They are associated with a specific organ system or meridian and they have inherent qualities that have a very powerful impact upon that organ itself. These flavors can help create balance within the body and can also help to bring a person into harmony with the seasons. It is also important to note that too much of a specific flavor can also do harm to its corresponding organ system. For example sweet foods can help to tonify the spleen/stomach and improve digestive function, but too much sweet foods can result in weakening the digestive capacity and creating sugar imbalances like diabetes or metabolic syndrome.

1. Sour

2. Bitter

3. Sweet

4. Acrid (spicy/pungent)

5. Salty

Additionally some people consider Bland to be a flavor, but this isn't directly associated with the five element theory, even though bland foods and herbs can be very beneficial and are associated with diuretic actions. Otherwise they are considered a division of the sweet flavor.

Organ System Association

In Chinese medicine the organ systems (zang-fu) are a detailed blue print of the makeup of the human form. The organ systems are not only the physiological tissue that comprises each vital organ but the entirety of its bio-mechanical pathways, mechanisms, and associations with nature such as emotion, taste, sense organ, season, color, and time.

The five flavors are directly linked with a specific organ system and each flavor helps to benefit its related organ system, but over consumption of a specific flavor can cause harm as well. Sour foods are associated with the liver and gallbladder (as well as the health of our tendons and ligaments), so too much sour food can cause injury or pain and cramping of our sinews. Bitter foods, such as coffee, are associated with the heart/small intestines organs in Chinese medicine and while coffee can stimulate fluid circulation and help increase your metabolism, too much can be overly drying on your body.

- Sour - Liver/gallbladder

- Bitter - Heart/small intestine

- Sweet - Spleen/stomach

- Acrid - Lung/large intestine

- Salty - Kidneys/bladder

Energetics and Therapeutic uses of the Five Flavors

- Sour: Astringents, helps to control Qi, blood, shen, essence. Helps retain our needed body fluids, moves inward and downward. Can help promote contraction in the digestive system.

- Bitter: Clears and purges, helps to dry dampness, consolidates yin, and calms shen, has desending movement.

- Sweet: Supplements, tonifies and moistens, reduces side effects of other herbs, lifting action, great choice when conditions of dryness are present, such as some conditions of constipation.

- Acrid: Causes upward and outward movement, dispersing, promotes Qi and blood circulation, lifting action.

- Salty: Energetically leads downwards and softens hardness, helps purge, can help lubricate intestines and help remove waste accumulation.

Examples of Foods Related to the Five Flavors

- Sour: Some examples are pomegranate, vinegar, lime, lemon, fermented foods.

- Bitter: Parsley, mustard greens, kale,dandelion greens, collard greens, burdock root, coffee.

- Sweet: Rice, chicken, whole grains, sweet potatoes, cabbage, carrots, onions, squashes, corn, fruits, goji berries, honey.

- Acrid: These foods include things like scallions, daikon radish, ginger.

- Salty: Seaweeds, miso, sea salt, tamari, pickles, ocean fish, shellfish.

Tips to Incorporate this Diet into your Life:

- Listen to your body: This is always number one. The best diet plan is one that works for the individuals unique needs and specific constitution.

- Seasonal eating: Eating according to the seasons is very important as our bodies also go through cyclical changes throughout the year. This is not only about eating fruits and vegetables that are currently in season, but following the five element examples of foods that can help bring you into balance.

- Eating at regular intervals: The earth element (spleen/stomach organ systems) loves a routine, so eating at regular times of the day can help assist the gastro-intestinal tract to perform optimally. And remember not to skip breakfast or eat more than you need.

- Eat moderate amounts: It is important to listen to your body when it tell you it is "full" or has had enough. Overeating makes it hard for the Spleen and Stomach to effectively digest food and allocate the nutrients to parts of the body that need it the most. Underrating may leave the body malnourished or dehydrated leading to things such as constipation or slow healing times.

- Make breakfast your largest meal: The first meal of the day helps to ignite your digestive system and the morning hours are also the time when the organs of the digestive system are most active according to the Chinese medicine clock (stomach 7-9 am and spleen 9-11 am).

- Cut back in the cold raw foods: Too much cold foods can slow down our physiological processes, and create dampness, and out out our digestive fires, so a Chinese diet tends to stay away from things like ice water, smoothies and too many raw salads. Opt for room temperature water, slightly steamed vegetables, and if you are craving those crunchy raw salads, have a cup of nice warm soup or bone broth first. Go easy on damp creating foods such as dairy, fatty foods, refined sugars, which can slow down your metabolism and the spleen and stomachs process of transformation and transportation, and may lead to sluggish activity of the Liver.

- Eat lots of veggies: Pretty simple advice- fill your plate with mainly fresh lightly cooked vegetables, your body will thank you.

- Cook and eat mindfully: Taking time to cook and eat is important, so slow down, turn off your phone and chew your food fully. Mindfulness can help boost your digestion, turn around any unwanted relationships around food and make you feel better all around. This new awareness can also help you tune in to any food sensitivities or foods that may not be best for your body. Try to avoid eating when you are stressed-out or aggravated as this can negatively impact digestion.

- Get up and move: In Chinese medicine the root of many diseases is stagnation, and lack of movement and Qi flow, so make sure you get your blood moving. Daily exercise can help boost your metabolism and improve your digestive function.

References

- Many-benefits-chinese-cupping, news: pacificcollege.edu, Retrieved 23 June, 2019
- Tuina, health: healthline.com, Retrieved 12 April, 2019
- Gua-sha benefits, health: healthline.com, Retrieved 17 March, 2019
- The-benefits-of-acupressure: verywellhealth.com, Retrieved 3 May, 2019
- Art, tai-chi, in-depth, stress-management, healthy-lifestyle: mayoclinic.org, Retrieved 21 March , 2019
- Chinese-medicine-diet-recommendations: wildearthacupuncture.com, Retrieved 13 June, 2019

Permissions

Index